> FULLY REVISED AND UPDATED

Bicycling MAGAZINE'S

**Greater Power,
Faster Speed,
Longer Endurance,
Better Skills**

TRAINING TECHNIQUES FOR CYCLISTS

EDITED BY BEN HEWITT

RODALE

© 2005 by Rodale Inc.

Rodale books may be purchased for business or promotional use or for special sales. For information, please write to: Special Markets Departments, Rodale Inc., 733 Third Avenue, New York, NY 10017

Bicycling is a registered trademark of Rodale Inc.

Printed in the United States of America
Rodale Inc. makes every effort to use acid-free ∞, recycled paper ♻.

Cover photograph by © John Kelly/Getty Images
Interior photographs by Jim Cummins/CORBIS,
Alan Jakubek/CORBIS, Pete Saloutos/CORBIS

Book design by Drew Frantzen

Portions of this book were originally published as *Bicycling® Magazine's Training Techniques for Cyclists* by Rodale Inc. © 1999.

Library of Congress Cataloging-in-Publication Data

Bicycling magazine's training techniques for cyclists : greater power, faster speed, longer endurance, better skills / edited by Ben Hewitt.— Fully rev. and updated.
    p.   cm.
Includes index.
ISBN-13 978–1–59486–052–2 paperback
ISBN-10 1–59486–052–1 paperback
    1. Cycling—Training. I. Title: Training techniques for cyclists. II. Hewitt, Ben,
date. III. Bicycling.
GV1048.B53   2005
796.6—dc22
    2005000597

Distributed to the book trade by Holtzbrinck Publishers

    4   6   8   10   9   7   5   3   paperback

We inspire and enable people to improve their lives and the world around them
For more of our products visit rodalestore.com or call 800-848-4735

CONTENTS

INTRODUCTION

If you've opened this book, you want to ride your bike faster. Period. It's a clear, simple desire, and it's probably been with you for decades, ever since you took that first, wobbly roll down the driveway on your first two-wheeler.

But that's where the clarity and simplicity end because to call cycling training "complex" would be an understatement of epic proportions. There are numerous reasons for this, but the primary one is this: No two cyclists are exactly alike. Every cyclist's body—and mind—reacts uniquely to training techniques, intensities, and loads. Bearing in mind varying goals (road race, criterium, time trial), styles (mountain, road, cyclocross), and levels of development (beginner to seasoned pro), you can begin to understand why there is no such thing as a universal training program.

Of course, crafting a training program that's as unique as your cycling is part of the fun. It's a craft made somewhat easier by training truths that are, if not universal, then nearly so. The goal of this book is to present these truths in an easy-to-understand manner and offer some suggestions for implementing them into your riding routine.

As you read this book, do so with an open mind and a willingness to experiment. Some techniques may work well for you; some may not. But rest assured: If you commit to structuring your training based on at least some of the concepts outlined in the following pages, you *will* ride faster. It's as clear and simple as that.

1

IN THE BEGINNING

You're fired up, ready to climb every mountain, sprint for every town limit sign, and bomb down every root-strewn descent. Excellent. Motivation is a critical, often overlooked component of a successful training program (we'll talk a lot more about that later). But before you leap off the sofa and into your Lycra, we need to go over a few things. It won't take long, and I'll try to make it as painless as possible.

Concept #1: To ride faster, you need to ride faster.

I know what you're thinking: "Well, duh." Yet you'd be surprised how many cyclists simply grind out hour after hour at, say, 16 mph, expecting that they'll magically be able to turn it up to 20 mph on the day of the local AIDS ride or citizens' race. To those riders, I have three words for you: Ain't gonna happen. Oh, sure, you'll make the first few miles okay; but soon your muscles, unaccustomed to the increased intensity, will be overrun with lactic acid and grind to a screechingly painful halt. Ultimately, you'll be lucky to average even your normal 16 mph pace.

So, it's clear: If you want to be able to ride 20 mph on the big day, you have to be able to ride 20 mph on the smaller days, too. In fact, you should be able to ride even faster than your goal pace, which sounds sort of mean until you realize that you needn't, nor should you, ride that speed for very long. The concept is similar to that of vaccines: By introducing your body to a controlled amount of something that can be very bad for you (in this case, super-high intensity), you're able to handle the lower intensities without cracking.

Concept #2: To ride faster, you need to ride slower.

I know what you're thinking: "What the heck's wrong with this guy? He just told me that to ride faster, I need to ride faster. That makes sense. Now he's telling me that to ride faster, I need to ride slower. What's he been putting in his water bottle?"

I agree; it defies logic. But it is imperative that you believe me at least enough to keep reading.

There are two reasons that most of your riding time (as much as 80 percent) should be spent at a pace far below that which you're trying to achieve. For one, your body and mind simply can't handle large volumes of high-intensity training. We'll discuss the physiological reasons for this later, but for now, trust me: If you train too hard too often, you'll actually get *slower*. Not good. For another, low-intensity training actually increases the body's capacity to handle higher paces. Again, we'll discuss this in greater detail later on; for now, file this little nugget under Perhaps the Most Important Thing Anyone Ever Told Me about Training.

Okay. Now you know 99 percent more than 99 percent of cyclists know about training. But the real trick—and the reason the remaining pages of this book exist—is seamlessly combining these diametrically opposed concepts into a cohesive training program. And to do that, there are a few more things you need to know. Read on.

The Language of Training

As you dig into this book, you're going to come across words and phrases that may be foreign to you. And even if you've heard them, you may not be entirely sure what they mean or how they fit in the context of cycling. Endurance training has a language all its own; to help you learn how to read and speak it, let's tackle some of the key terms and concepts.

Aerobic Capacity

Also known as max VO$_2$, aerobic capacity is the measure of how much oxygen your body can use during maximal exertion. Obviously, the higher your aerobic capacity, the better. Improved aerobic capacity is one of the major goals of training; but it must be noted that while training can increase aerobic capacity (AC), genetics plays a leading role in determining its boundaries. In other words, pick your parents well. And don't age: Aerobic capacity drops by an estimated 1 percent per year after age 25, though individuals who exercise regularly can reduce that decline significantly.

Anaerobic Threshold

Otherwise known as lactate threshold, the anaerobic threshold (AT) is the level of exertion at which lactic acid begins to accumulate in the blood. That searing pain in your quads during hard efforts? That's lactic acid at work. Accumulate enough lactic acid, and you'll have no choice but to slow down. However, unlike your aerobic capacity, your AT is highly trainable. In other words, smart training can raise it significantly, allowing you to ride at a higher percentage of your maximal ability. In fact, while sedentary folks have an AT that's about 50 percent of their AC, highly trained athletes boast ATs that run about 90 percent of AC. That's why AC is not a very good predictor of performance; just because someone has a high AC doesn't mean that they can work to its potential.

Frequency

This one's pretty simple: how often you do a training session. What's really important to understand is that frequency is a relative term. For a new rider, training four times per week might represent an appropriate frequency, while more experienced riders might train that often in 2 days by performing "two-a-days." The frequency at which you train should be based on your current level of development.

Duration

Again, pretty easy: the length of your training sessions. Obviously, this is largely dependent on your current state of development and your goals for the particular workout. An experienced racer training for a long road race might do regular 4- and 5-hour rides, while a Category 4 criterium racer's program will focus on training rides of much shorter duration.

Volume

Add your frequency and duration, and you get volume, your total training load measured in hours. It's tempting to focus on volume simply because it's so easy to determine. But in and of itself, volume is not a very good indicator of training quality. That's because it ignores:

Intensity

Intensity is the single biggest factor in determining an athlete's success (or lack thereof). Intensity is sort of like salt in a recipe: Get the right amount, and it makes your food sing. But too little or too much, and you'll be pushing your plate away after only a few bites. Consequently, training intensity is the ingredient most riders get wrong. They go either too hard, too often, not hard enough, not often enough, or any combination of the four.

Overtraining

Defined as a condition of lackluster performance resulting from too much volume, intensity, or both, overtraining is the black hole of cycling and has ended many a season (and career) prematurely. Overtraining can be hard to diagnose simply because its symptoms can mimic the opposite cause: undertraining. Most cyclists figure that if they're not riding well, it must be because they're undertrained. In some cases, that's true; but in many, many more, it's overtraining, not undertraining, that's the cause of their woe.

Overload

Overload differs from overtraining in that it's a conscious, even desirable, condition brought on by a short period of intense training designed to stimulate the body into adaptation to higher stress levels. A successful training program repeats an overload-recovery-adaptation-overload cycle that consistently ratchets up fitness. It's critical to understand that overload is merely the catalyst for performance improvement; without adequate recovery, the body will not have an opportunity to adapt, and performance will actually decline.

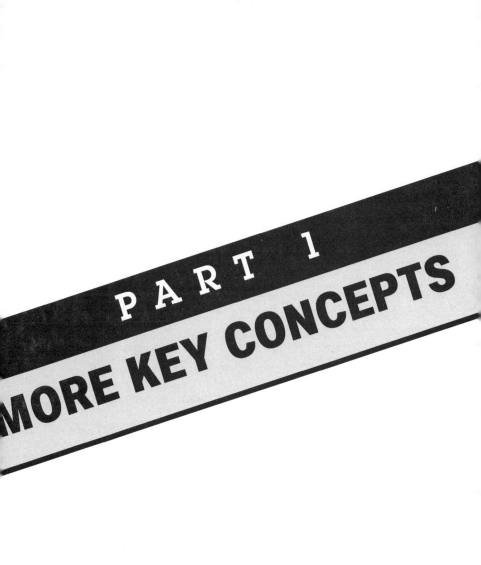

PART 1

MORE KEY CONCEPTS

2

PEDALING LIKE A PRO

When Lance Armstrong emerged from the shadows of cancer to win his first Tour de France, people were stunned. He was a rider transformed both in body and technique. The cancer and resultant chemotherapy took care of the former; Armstrong and coach Chris Carmichael handled the latter.

Most noticeable was Armstrong's newfound pedaling style. All pros look enviably supple and smooth on the bike (hey, if you rode 20,000 miles a year, you'd look pretty darn good on a bike, too), but Armstrong had taken it up a notch: While his competition maintained cadences (pedal rotation) that ranged between 80 and 90 rotations per minute (and often much less on steep climbs), Armstrong floated down the road with his pedals turning a hummingbird-like 100 to 110 rpm. And when he hit the mountains, his cadence barely slowed.

Pedaling is so integral to being a strong, efficient rider that you must address it before moving on to actual training techniques. Too many cyclists take pedaling for granted, thinking that it's just a matter of making their legs go up and down. While an efficient pedaling stroke can't actually make you fitter, it can maximize the fitness you do have. Think of it as free speed. Ah, now we have your attention.

Counting Cadence

Cadence is a simple measure of leg speed, not unlike the tachometer in your car. And just as your car runs most efficiently at certain rpm, so too does your body. Next time you're out and about, take a look at the pedaling style of occasional riders (they're typically wearing jeans and no helmet). Most grind along in a high gear, turning the pedals at 40 or 50 rpm. This is partly because to someone who hasn't trained their legs to rotate faster, this pace feels normal. And it's due partly to a misguided belief that the way to go faster is to push a bigger gear.

Well, they're wrong. If you're training for fitness and possibly competition, your pedaling cadence should average at least 80 rpm and go as high as the 100 to 110 rpm Armstrong employs. Maintaining this brisk sort of cadence is called *spinning*, which rhymes with winning, which means we like it.

To monitor your cadence while riding, simply count the number of times one foot comes through its pedal stroke (count at the top or the bottom of the stroke) over the course of 30 seconds and multiply by 2. The result is your pedaling rpm. You can also purchase a cyclecomputer, which will provide a constant, real-time cadence display. In either case, you should monitor your cadence on a variety of terrains, including climbs, flats, and descents. It will certainly vary, but try to keep your climbing cadence within 15 percent of your rpm on the flats (if you're maintaining 100 rpm on the flats, shoot for 85 rpm when climbing). You probably won't be able to keep the gap this close at first. In fact, you'll probably be quite frustrated to find that you're suddenly climbing in a lower gear and going slower up the hills. But as your body becomes accustomed to the increased pedal speed, you'll soon be riding faster, with more energy in reserve.

Why? First, riding fast requires a high rate of work, and you're simply more efficient at a high cadence. By spinning moderate gears instead of grinding bigger ones to maintain a given speed, your leg muscles stay fresher and allow you to train more effectively. A good analogy is lifting weights: You could probably lift a 5-pound weight all day long. But if you added up the cumulative weight lifted and tried to heft it all at once, you wouldn't be able to budge it. That's an extreme example, but the theory is exactly the same. The faster you spin, the less force is required to move the pedals and the more you're dividing the work load into smaller, more manageable chunks.

Second, and of utmost concern to racers, a high cadence facilitates rapid acceleration. Again, let's use the car analogy: When you're setting up to pass on a short stretch of two-lane highway, what's the first thing you do? Shift to a lower gear, which increases engine rpm and gives you greater acceleration. The same goes for pedaling a bicycle. Spinning lower gears allows you to react much more quickly to rapid changes in speed, such as when a competitor attacks. Rather than finding yourself bogged down in too high a gear, you'll be able to match his effort, get on his wheel, and, of course, beat him to the finish line.

Finally, spinning is easier on the knees. Churning a big gear loads these delicate hinges beyond their capacities, and you can end up with debilitating injuries. That, in short, is a very bad thing.

Finding Your Perfect Cadence

Your ideal cadence depends on your type of riding. During criteriums, which are typically run over flat roads and feature lots of corners and constant attacks from rivals, you'll want to maintain a very high cadence for quick acceleration out of the corners and to respond to attacks. Shoot for 90 to 100 rpm.

Conversely, time trialists need not worry about attacks or sudden changes of pace and might find a slightly lower cadence (say, 80 rpm) more suited to this powerful riding style. Mountain bikers will typically find themselves pedaling at these relatively low cadences, too. That's because a high cadence can cause a rider to get bounced around a lot on the roots, rocks, and uneven terrain common to off-road riding.

Long-distance road racers and fit recreational cyclists should borrow from each of these styles in search of the cadence that feels and works best for them. These riders should avoid marrying themselves to a particular number and instead should let their bodies be the guide. But remember: If you've been grinding out the low-cadence, high-gear miles, spinning is going to feel strange. Give your body time to adapt.

If you want to get scientific, you can borrow a technique from Lance Armstrong, who used a heart-rate monitor to help determine the most efficient cadence for his purposes. To do this, you'll need to conduct several 10-minute time trials (ideally at least 2 days apart so you're fully rested) on both flat and climbing courses. Monitor your heart rate and average speed, using different gears to produce different cadences. Your optimal cadence is the one that produces the lowest heart rate and the highest speed. Keep in mind, however, that this test won't account for your body's future adaptation to a higher cadence, so if you're just starting down the path to spinning enlightenment, it's worth repeating this exercise monthly to see how the results differ.

3 »»»

KEYS TO BETTER PEDALING

There are some techniques you can utilize to make the transition to spinning smoother and more natural.

Get your saddle height right. You simply can't spin efficiently if your saddle is too high or too low. To check yours, measure your inseam length from crotch to floor while wearing socks. Hold the tape tight against your body (it may help to hook it over a stick) and stand with your feet 6 inches apart. Multiply the resulting number by 0.883. This should be the distance between the center of the bottom bracket axle (the very center of the crank arm, where it connects to the bottom bracket spindle) and the top of the seat, measured in a line with the bike's seat tube. While the 0.883 number sounds very precise, use this as a starting point, and don't be afraid to adjust your saddle height up or down from this position. Just be very aware of how these changes affect your pedaling style and, more important, how they affect your body.

Wipe your shoes. Thanks to Greg LeMond, an entire generation of riders has grown up with the shoe-scraping technique the champion cyclist recommends. As your foot and pedal come through the bottom of the pedal stroke, image you're scraping mud or (if you live in, say, Maine) snow off the bottom of your foot. This helps keep your heel high and eliminate the "dead spot" at the bottom of the pedal stroke.

Raise your knees. It's pretty much impossible to actually pull your pedals up when you're spinning at a good clip. But you can lighten the load on the upward pedal so that there's less weight for the opposite leg to push downward. World-champion mountain bike racer Ned Overend accomplishes this by visualizing his knees driving toward the handlebar. This helps pull his pedals up the back side and across the top of the stroke, another potential dead spot.

Ride rollers. Indoor trainers, which clamp your bike securely, may seem like the sane, safe choice. But the pros know that nothing refines your pedaling technique like rollers, which utilize free-rolling drums and force a gracefully smooth and balanced riding style, lest you come crashing down. Begin by riding in a doorway or next to a wall so you have something to hold until you become comfortable.

Ride a fixed gear. "Fixed gear" means that the rear cog is threaded directly onto the wheel; there's no freewheel mechanism. When the wheel turns, the pedals turn and, by extension, so do your legs (assuming they're attached to the pedals—if they're not, you really need to rethink your riding position). Mastering a fixed gear bike is particularly difficult, but neophyte fixed gear riders should not venture into city traffic, or carnage will almost certainly ensue. You can build up a spare fixed gear bike or have your current steed equipped. Check with your local bike shop for assistance.

Spin the descents. When the road points down, it's always tempting to drop into a big gear and go like the wind. But once in a while, keep your bike in a relatively low gear and boost your cadence to 120 or even more. Try to relax and concentrate on keeping your hips and upper body still as your legs whip around.

Target Training Intensities

This is where things get a bit more technical. But it's also where you stand to gain the greatest understanding of training theory—understanding that will lead you to the greatest fitness gains in the least time.

Let's say you ride six times each week for a total of 11 hours. Your best cycling buddy rides four times per week, logging only 7 hours. Who is improving their fitness more?

The answer is not as simple as it seems. In fact, your friend could be making significantly more progress. The reason lies in what those numbers don't tell—how hard each of you is riding. And, perhaps more importantly, how hard each of you is *resting*. Along with frequency and duration, intensity (or lack thereof) is an essential component in determining the effectiveness of training rides.

Here's the rub: While the number and length of rides are easily determined, intensity is more difficult to gauge. To measure it, you must know the amount of effort you're using, compared with the maximum you could generate if you were working at your full capacity.

The easiest, and most popular, method of gauging intensity is heart rate, which climbs in direct correlation to effort. When you're sleeping, it's very low. When you're sprinting up a climb with a pack of rabid wolves chasing, it's very, very high. In between are all the intensities of life and training. During an average ride, your heart rate usually fluctuates through a wide range but is almost always below 100 percent of maximum. The percentage of maximum accurately reflects your exercise intensity. For example, if your heart rate is at 80 percent of maximum, you're riding at 80 percent intensity.

Most exercise physiologists agree that to significantly improve fitness, you must maintain an intensity level of at least 65 percent. That's not to say your heart should *always* be thumping at 65 percent (or greater) of its maximum; in fact, there are important benefits to riding below this level. But if you want to get faster, you'll need to exceed 65 percent at least some of the time. By how much and how often is a much thornier subject, and we'll discuss it in greater detail later.

Find Your Maximum

Before you can attach a specific heart rate to 65 percent, you need to know what 100 percent is. There are several ways, with varying accuracy. Perhaps the most accurate is to take a medical stress test. This is a grand idea, especially if you're returning to exercise after a sedentary period. But these tests are expensive and time-consuming, so you may want to consider one of the following two alternatives.

The first is a simple formula: Subtract your age from 220. If you're 40, for instance, the result is 180, your theoretical maximum heart rate. But beware: This formula is notoriously inaccurate, by as much as 15 beats per minute (bpm) in either direction. That's more than enough to send you down a path of over- (or under-) training.

A better (but decidedly more arduous) method is to use a long, steep hill and wireless heart-rate monitor (good ones, which transmit via chest strap, start at about $75). Perform your maximum heart rate test on a day when you're well-rested; you should have done only easy rides for at least the previous 2 days. Warm up for at least 15 minutes, and start the climb at a steady tempo, slowly bringing your heart rate up until it feels like you can't go any faster. At this point, sprint like the hounds of hell were on your trail. The number flashing on your heart-rate monitor when you are forced to back off will be your maximum, or quite nearly so (most people are able to push their heart rates a few beats higher during competition, but the number you get during this test is accurate enough to base your training on).

But perhaps more critical to determining training intensity is your anaerobic or lactate threshold (we'll go with anaerobic and use "AT"), the point at which your muscles become overwhelmed by lactic acid and you're forced to back off. Your AT is the marker on which you're going to base your hard training because more than anything else, riding fast means being able to sustain AT efforts. Too, proper training will actually raise your AT, which means you'll be able to ride faster before blowing up. Or throwing up.

Note: Before subjecting yourself to the exertion of a maximum heart rate test, get your doctor's approval. This is especially important if you are over 35, overweight, or sedentary or have a family history of cardiac problems.

Determine Your AT

To determine your AT, you need a heart-rate monitor that tracks average heart rate and a stretch of flat or gradually uphill road that will take you 30 minutes to ride all-out. Plan your AT test for a day when you're well-rested; you should abstain from hard training for at least 2 days prior.

Warm up for at least 20 minutes before beginning the test. Throw in a couple of 1- to 2-minute efforts toward the end of the warmup to wake up your legs, and be sure to arrive at the "start line" of your test loose, limber, and sweating lightly.

Hit the stopwatch on your heart-rate monitor and start pedaling. Try to settle into a comfortable rhythm as quickly as possible, remembering to maintain a pace you can hold for 30 minutes. In other words, don't go out too hard. After 10 minutes, hit the lap button on your monitor (if you don't have one, restart your monitor); the average heart rate for the final 20 minutes of your ride is an excellent indicator of your AT. Commit that number to memory. You're going to use it a whole bunch.

The Fat Myth

You've probably read somewhere that you burn more fat with low-intensity exercise. While it's true that at low intensities fat provides a higher percentage of fuel, it's also true that you lose weight by burning calories. And you'll burn more calories by riding harder.

For example, cycling for 1 hour at a heart rate of 120 bpm may burn 350 calories. Of these, about half (175) will be fat. Conversely, if you pedal harder and get your heart rate up to 160 bpm, you might burn as much as 1,000 calories during that same hour-long ride. At this intensity, only about one-fifth (200) of the calories will be from fat (still 25 more than at the lower intensity), but the calorie deficit created is much, much higher, meaning you're that much further along the path to losing weight (for each pound lost, you'll need to burn 3,500 calories).

This is doubly significant because of the way your body restocks calories. Studies show that when you exercise at low intensities and burn a high percentage of fat calories, your body replenishes these first. So, you end up right back where you started. If you're trying to lose weight, it's best to ride at the highest level that's sustainable and won't disrupt your training program. Don't restrict intensity in the mistaken belief that it's necessary in order to burn more fat. Likewise, don't sacrifice your training goals by riding too hard in an effort to burn more calories. Remember: There are very few overweight competitive cyclists. If you're riding enough to become competitive, you're riding enough that assuming a sensible diet, you're going to lose weight. It's one of the great perks of being a bike racer.

The Last Word on Intensity

There's no doubt that the only way to get fast is to ride fast. But there's a point of diminishing returns, and that point comes a lot quicker than you might think. Training at high intensities is very stressful to your body. That stress is good if it's carefully monitored and doled out in a structured form. But if you're not careful, it can literally ruin you as a cyclist. When in doubt, ride *easier* than you think you should be. You might sacrifice ultimate top-end fitness, but a slightly less fit but physically and mentally fresh cyclist will beat a super-fit but teetering-on-the-edge-of-burnout cyclist every time.

When in doubt, remember this: You actually get faster during periods of rest. That's because hard training breaks down—literally tears—muscle fibers. Then, during rest, they rebuild themselves to withstand even greater force. If you never rest, they'll never have a chance to rebuild, and you'll never get faster.

4

POWER TRAINING

Although using heart rate as an intensity gauge is better than using no gauge at all, it's not without its flaws. That's because your heart rate is influenced by numerous factors other than exercise: Stress, illness, and caffeine all wreak havoc on your ticker and can mean you're getting a false measure of intensity.

That's why many professional and elite amateur cyclists have turned to power as their primary method for measuring intensity and structuring workouts. While heart rate is simply an indicator of intensity, power—expressed as watts—is a direct representation of how hard you are pedaling. For instance, while caffeine can raise your heart rate at a given exertion level, you can drink as much coffee as you want, and 200 watts will still be 200 watts.

Power is also useful because going fast on a bicycle, especially up hills, is all about maximizing your power-to-weight ratio. Here's an example: You weigh 170 pounds and can generate an average of 320 watts during a 20-minute climb. Your chief rival can generate only 290 watts. But he weighs only 140 pounds. Who's going to hit the top first? All things (equipment, weather conditions, mental preparedness) being equal, you're gonna get beat. That's because you're generating 1.88 watts per pound, to his 2.07. His power-to-weight ratio is higher, which means he'll climb faster.

How do you improve your power-to-weight ratio? Well, you can increase your power output through training (if you'd been able to produce 360 watts in the above example, you would've been the champ). And you can lose weight (if you could dump 20 pounds and still maintain 320 watts, your watts per pound would climb to 2.13, enough to leave your rival gasping in your dust). Power-to-weight ratio is why committed pros like Lance Armstrong are fanatical about their diets (Armstrong is famous for weighing every morsel of food that passes his lips, in order to get an accurate calorie count). At the highest levels of cycling, where climbs last for upwards of an hour and come five or six to the stage, a loss of only 2 or 3 pounds can prove critical.

But there's a delicate balance between power and weight. Lose too much weight, and you'll begin to lose muscle mass and, therefore, power. The key is keeping power levels high (through careful training and diet) while maximizing healthy weight loss. For most amateur cyclists, weighing their food and fretting over every last calorie simply isn't worth the hassle. Too, the climbs we scale simply aren't as arduous as the big European mountains. Power to weight is still a big deal, but it's not the end-all, be-all factor.

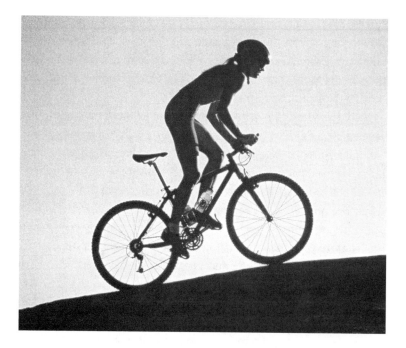

Which raises the question: Should you train with a power meter? Ideally, yes. But there's yet another factor to consider: Power meters are enormously expensive. Reliable models start at $800, with full-featured units running well into the thousands. For the professional or committed amateur, it's money well-spent. The rest of us should take a close look at our goals (and bank accounts) before jumping.

Too Much Information?

There's another take on power meters, and it comes from Rick Crawford, a cycling coach based in Durango, Colorado, who counts Olympic mountain biker Todd Wells and rising road star Tom Danielson among his clients: "The information overload that modern athletes have access to has dulled perception," says Crawford. "From a coaching standpoint, I love the numbers. But if I could have one tool, it'd be perception. I don't want my athlete to be crippled when they don't have numbers."

For that reason, says Crawford, cyclists need to exercise caution when using any of the newfangled training devices. "A lot of kids know that Lance Armstrong does 400 watts, so they'll go out and kill themselves to do 400 watts, even though it's a number that has no bearing on their optimal training."

Still, Crawford thinks power meters can be an important tool for serious cyclists. "Power meters give us an absolute measure of performance; it's the best barometer of fitness because it eliminates guesswork and environmental factors." For this reason, Crawford likes to use power meters to gauge an athlete's progress as the season unfolds. The problem comes when eager cyclists forgo daily perception and other measures to focus solely on power. "In many ways, heart rate is more valuable information precisely *because* it's subjective," says Crawford. "It's the little nuances that can tell an alert rider when to back off and when to push harder."

The upshot? The information provided by heart-rate monitors and power meters can greatly benefit your training and improve your performance. There's no doubt about that. But it must be taken in context. And it should never become the sole focus of your training. "There's nothing sadder than a cyclist out on a lonely road, just staring at the numbers," says Crawford. "Not only is it not fun, but no one's giving out sponsorships for power meter and heart-rate monitor downloads. Don't live in numbers."

Perceived Exertion

So, what's the alternative? It's simple, really: how hard you feel like you're going. It's called perceived exertion or rate of perceived exertion (RPE), and it's an admittedly subjective assessment of your effort.

Still, this is one of the best tools you can have in your workshop of training. In fact, many highly experienced athletes prefer to rely solely on perceived exertion. For the beginning competitor, this isn't a good idea, but when combined with hard numbers from a heart-rate monitor, cyclecomputer, or power meter, RPE is a critical piece of information.

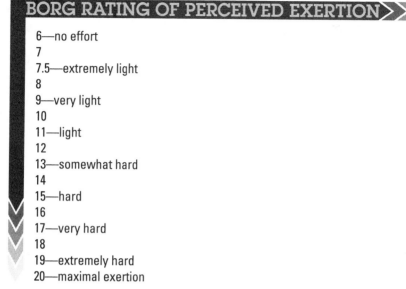

BORG RATING OF PERCEIVED EXERTION >>>>

6—no effort
7
7.5—extremely light
8
9—very light
10
11—light
12
13—somewhat hard
14
15—hard
16
17—very hard
18
19—extremely hard
20—maximal exertion

To understand how RPE works, take a look at the Borg Rating of Perceived Exertion, which rates effort on a scale of 6 to 20.

For a cyclist's purposes, anything under 10 should be considered recovery; 10–12 is where aerobic development occurs and where you should complete endurance rides; 13–14 is where muscular endurance and force begin to blossom; 15–16 is just below your AT, where you'll start to develop race-level fitness; 17 is right at the AT; and anything above should be held in reserve for competition or carefully metered interval training (more on this later).

5 >> >> >>

OVERTRAINING

Whether cyclists use a heart-rate monitor, a power meter, or simple instinct to monitor their workouts, they run the risk of overtraining. "But not me," you say. "I only ride 5 or 6 hours a week. How can I overtrain?"

The answer is, quite easily. That's because it's the total stress in your life that leads to overtraining, not just cycling stress. As far as your body and mind are concerned, cycling is just one more stress heaped on top of all the others. Are you trying to fit those 5 riding hours in around a 60-hour workweek and family obligations? Are you losing sleep to squeeze in training rides? Are you losing sleep because you can't squeeze in training rides?

Yes, pro cyclists routinely ride 25 hours—or more—each week. But that's all they do. And they're supported in a way amateurs can only dream of: daily massages, naps, careful food preparation. Contrast that to your schedule. If you're like most amateur cyclists, you work at least 40 hours each week, ride herd on the kids, juggle a budget, mow the lawn, clean the gutters, take the pets to the vet, and . . . You get the picture.

The key to managing your stress and avoiding overtraining is to make sure riding your bicycle is a stress reducer, not increaser. As soon as you start stressing out over your training, back off. This is exactly when you're most prone to sickness, burnout, and the spiraling black hole of overtraining.

Depths of Fatigue

Cycling is a tough sport; to get better, you're going to have to get tired. But you need to learn how to discern between the cycling-specific fatigue you feel the day after a race or a hard workout and the systemic fatigue that's often the first warning sign of overtraining.

One of the first signs of overtraining is an elevated resting heart rate. Get in the habit of checking your heart rate when you first wake up, before you get out of bed. Do this for 10 days straight, and write the numbers down. On the 10th day, find the average. This is your resting heart rate, and you should continue to monitor it, particularly during periods of intense training. If it jumps by 10 percent or more, consider yourself warned: Your body is telling you to back off. Listen to it.

Other indications of overtraining include:

Nagging ailments. If you catch successive colds, suspect overtraining. Studies have shown that your immune system is compromised during periods of high stress, and upper-respiratory infections are often the result. Another signal is that saddle sores and minor wounds are slow to heal.

Lingering soreness. Once you're accustomed to cycling, you should experience little muscle soreness, even after hard days. That's because cycling is a non-weight-bearing sport and, as such, is relatively easy on the muscles and joints. Your legs might feel a bit tight and sore after a tough day, but any discomfort should disappear relatively quickly. If it lingers longer than 48 hours, take a couple of days off.

Stagnant performance. Every cyclist experiences bad days, when it feels like they can't ride their way out of a paper bag. One of the worst mistakes you can make is to push your way through a bad day, forcing your body to go harder than it wants to. If after a couple of efforts you simply can't click the gears over like usual, back off. Likewise, if you're unable to get your heart rate or power up to typical levels, ease up. Resting will be of far greater benefit.

Disposition. While this may seem the vaguest possible index, it's actually one of the most reliable. In one study involving swimmers, measurements of such things as anger, depression, and vigor worsened markedly when training loads were doubled. Put simply, if you're in a crappy mood all the time, take some time off the bike. Apathy is another warning sign. If you used to get fired up just thinking about riding but now can't drag yourself off the couch, you're probably overtrained.

Bouncing Back

Okay. So you're overtrained. Now what? There's only one cure, and you're not going to like it: rest. You need to coddle your abused body and nurse it back to health. Plan on hanging up the bike for at least a week, and when you come back to it, do only easy rides for at least another 10 days. If you're afraid of losing fitness, consider this: Whatever fitness lost won't be half as much as the fitness you'll lose if you try to train through it. In fact, many a cyclist has lost an entire season to overtraining by not recognizing and heeding the warning signs.

To speed recovery, try to get a massage or two, which helps flush the muscles of unwanted metabolic by-products and also helps relax you, physically and mentally. Pay particular attention to eating a nutritious diet, but don't stress out over it. Stress is what got you into this fix in the first place; do everything you can to avoid it.

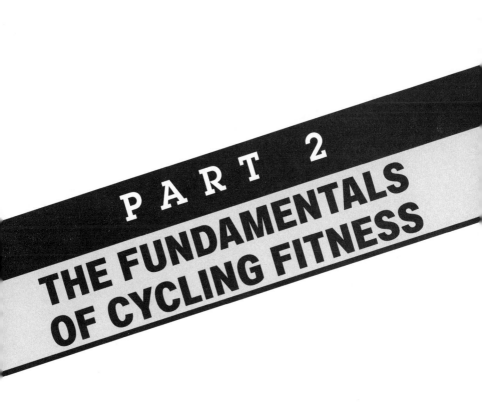

PART 2

THE FUNDAMENTALS OF CYCLING FITNESS

Y ou can do a lot of different things on a bicycle. You can ride fast. You can ride far. You can ride on road or off, uphill or down. You can sprint. Ideally, you'd be able to do every one of these things well. Problem is, training for improvement in some departments can actually impede your ability in others. For instance, most riders are either strong time trialists or climbers. That's because the best climbers tend to be lithe, while the best time trialists tend to have powerful, muscular builds. Few riders can ride both disciplines at a truly elite level, which is why only a handful of cyclists are capable of winning the Tour de France, which demands world-beating climbing and time trialing fitness.

Therefore, before we go any further, you need to make an honest assessment of your abilities and goals. First, take moment and think about what you want to accomplish with your training. Maybe you want to someday race the Tour de France, or perhaps you simply want to finish a local mountain bike race. Does the speed of criterium racing get your blood going? Or maybe you don't want to race at all; for you, group charity rides sound like fun.

Once you've determined your goals, it's time to take a look at your limitations as a cyclist. (warning: humbling ahead). If you've been riding awhile, you probably know what your strengths and weaknesses are, but if you're new to the sport, it might seem like *everything* is a weakness. To a certain extent, that's true, but there are two fairly accurate predictors to what you'll be good at. The first is body type. Are you taking up cycling after an NFL career? Then you'll probably make a better sprinter or crit rider than climber. On the other hand, if you're 6 feet tall and 140 pounds dripping wet, look to the mountains because that's where you'll be able to press the advantage of your beanpole build. The other is simple desire. If you *want* to be a climber, if that's what gets you psyched to swing a leg over your saddle each morning, chances are you'll become a good, or at least decent, climber, even if your body type says "no."

If you're reading this book solely because you want to win races, it makes sense to pick a discipline that suits your body type. Basically, that means that if you're wide-shouldered and generally big-boned, you should look to crits and time trials. And if you have trouble walking a straight line in a stiff breeze? Consider road and cross-country mountain bike racing. But remember (and this is especially true if you're new to endurance athletics): Body types change with training and a healthy diet. Put in enough miles and eat wisely, and you'll earn the lean physique of a professional cyclist.

Without further ado, let's take a look at the fundamentals of cycling fitness and where they come into play.

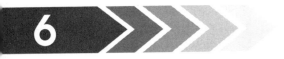

THE CYCLIST'S DIET

If you're feeling confused about nutrition, you're not alone. With all the conflicting advice going around, probably the only people who aren't confused are the ones who aren't paying attention. And given the hype surrounding the diet du jour, one wonders if perhaps they aren't better off for it.

That might be true if they weren't engaged in regular, rigorous physical activity. But as a serious cyclist, you demand more of your body than sedentary people. The food you put into your body is quite literally the fuel that powers your rides; you can't expect your body to run like a Ferrari if you're filling it up with low-octane gas.

Okay, but how do you know what's good for you and what's not? If you're tired of feeling perplexed—and perhaps bouncing from one fad diet to another, only to learn the hard way that radical eating plans, magic ingredients, and expensive supplements don't work, this chapter is for you. It contains all you need to know about eating for good health and better cycling performance. No hype. No promises. Just the facts.

The Case for Carbohydrates

These days, it seems as if you can't even lift a glass of orange juice in public without garnering dirty looks. It's as if you were lighting a cigar in the children's room of the local library. The current low-carb trend is intriguing, if only because it flies in the face of conventional cycling nutrition wisdom. For decades, sports nutritionists have been telling us to stuff our faces with pasta and potatoes and pancakes and . . . You get the idea. Basically, everything the mass media are now telling us we shouldn't eat.

So, where's the beef (or, perhaps more to the point, the bread)? Let's get one thing straight: Atkins was not a competitive cyclist. Carbohydrates are still your best bet for fueling your cycling escapades.

Why? "For any extended aerobic effort, you need carbohydrates for fuel and recovery," says Liz Applegate, Ph.D., author of *Eat Smart, Play Hard* and a professor at the University of California in Davis. "Cyclists who follow low-carb diets come to me all the time saying, 'You know, my legs just don't feel good.'" That's because during and after exercise, your body needs readily accessible fuel, and carbohydrate is more available to your muscles than protein or fat. It simply takes less energy to convert carbohydrate—which is essentially sugar—into usable fuel. Simple carbohydrate is a single or double sugar molecule—usually glucose, fructose, galactose, sucrose, or lactose. These are found in nutritious foods (such as fruit and dairy), as well as in less healthful fare, such as candy. Complex carbohydrate is a long chain of simple sugars and is often called a starch. Potatoes, pasta, and whole grain bread are good examples.

When you eat carbohydrate, it's broken down and converted to blood glucose, the body's main fuel and the only type that can feed the brain. Glucose that's not immediately used for energy is stored in the muscles and liver as glycogen and later used for fuel. If these spots are full, the glucose is converted to fat.

Yes, protein and fat can fuel your body and brain (if they couldn't, all those Atkins advocates would be in serious trouble). But the energy demands of cycling, especially at high intensities, simply can't be satisfied by this cumbersome process. That's why you need carbo-hydrate, and a heck of a lot more than the 50 grams per day suggested by some low-carb diets. In fact, Dr. Applegate recommends that people engaged in regular aerobic exercise consume 400 to 600 grams of carbohydrate daily.

All Carbs Are Not Created Equal

This is an important concept to grasp because it has a major impact on how your body responds to the carbohydrates you eat.

During and immediately after a hard ride, simple and complex car-bohydrates are equally effective as fuel. Your body is in a state of carbohydrate deficit (when you are exercising at high intensities, it's virtually impossible to replenish carbohydrate at the rate you're burning it), and it's critical to renew those stockpiles as quickly as possible for recovery's sake. But in your general diet, it's best to em-phasize the complex type of carbohydrate, for a number of reasons.

For one, complex carbs are typically accompanied by other impor-tant nutrients, such as vitamins, minerals, and fiber. Consider: A candy bar and whole grain bagel provide approximately the same number of calories, with approximately the same percentage of those calories taking the form of carbohydrate. But the candy bar is chock-full of what's known as "empty calories," calories that don't provide your body with any substantive nutritional value. The bagel, on the other hand, contains numerous trace minerals and fiber, things our body needs to run smoothly.

Overall, nutritionists recommend that at least 60 percent of your calories come from carbohydrate. For cyclists and other aerobic ath-letes, 65 percent is better, particularly in the hours before and after a big effort. Food packaging lists carbohydrate content as a percentage of daily calories, making your intake fairly easy to track, and there are calorie-count books available that include the calorie breakdown of every conceivable unpackaged food. To help you determine how many grams of carbohydrate you need each day, here's a simple formula based on the 65 percent number.

First, determine your total daily calorie requirement by multiplying your weight by 15. To this number, add 10 calories (men) or 8 calories (women) for each minute of cycling you do each day. The total is roughly the number of daily calories you need to maintain your weight. To lose weight, consume 500 fewer calories each day. You'll lose 1 pound per week, a safe and sustainable rate.

For example, a 150-pound man who does a 1-hour training ride would figure as follows: $150 \times 15 = 2,250$ calories + 600 calories (10 calories $\times$ 60 minutes) = 2,850 total calories. For this rider, 65 percent of total calories amounts to about 1,850 (2,850 total calories $\times$ 0.65 = 1,852.5). This is the number of carb calories he should eat daily. Because carbohydrate has 4 calories per gram, he can divide 1,850 by 4 to determine that he needs about 460 grams of carbohydrate per day (1,850 carb calories divided by 4 calories per gram = 462.5 grams of carbohydrate).

Don't become chained to the math. You ride a bike because it's fun; eating is fun, too. Don't make it into another stress. The point is that you should emphasize whole grain breads, high-quality dairy products, pasta, rice, potatoes, vegetables, and fruits. Remember that a food in its whole form (an apple, compared with apple juice; potatoes, compared with potato chips) will always provide superior nutrition, and remember to keep your total daily calorie consumption in line with your expenditure (or see page 29, if you're trying to lose weight).

Why Low Carb Works for Nonathletes

No doubt you know someone whose body has undergone a transformation under the guidance of the Atkins or a similar low-carb diet. The reason is for this is simple: "It's not just a reduced-carbohydrate diet; it's a reduced-calorie diet," explains Dr. Applegate. In other words, by eliminating carbohydrate from their diet, they've eliminated what was their primary source of calories. If they were consuming 2,000 calories per day pre-Atkins, and 60 percent of those calories came from carbohydrates, they were eating 1,200 calories' worth of carbs each day. By eliminating those, they've eliminated 1,200 daily calories, and although they'll replace some of those with protein and fat calories, it's very difficult to eat that much protein and fat in a day. Low-carb diets work because they're low calorie, not because they're low carb. That's not to say you shouldn't experiment with reduced-carbohydrate eating. Particularly if you normally eat a lot of simple carbs, a reduced-carb diet can help stabilize your blood sugar and quell your sweet tooth. "If Cheez-Its are a staple of your diet, then you should think about cutting some carbs," says Dr. Applegate. "But again, the idea is to replace them with other, smarter carbs that are more filling and will help you eat fewer calories."

Getting Carb Smart

Most cyclists know which foods contain high levels of carbohydrates and can differentiate between those that harbor complex carbs and those that are chock-full of simple sugars. Bagel, good; candy bar, bad, right?

Well, it's not quite that simple, and that's because of something known as the glycemic index. Remember that phrase, and if you ever need to impress a nutritionist at a party, start throwing it around. But first, you'd better know what it is.

The glycemic index (GI) is a ranking of carbohydrates according to their immediate effect on blood sugar levels. Carbohydrates that break down quickly during digestion (simple carbs) have the highest glycemic indexes. The blood glucose response is fast and high. Carbohydrates that break down slowly (complex carbs), releasing glucose gradually into the bloodstream, have low glycemic indexes.

That's all pretty easy to understand. But it gets more complicated when you start looking at some of the foods that are high on the GI. For instance, potatoes, a staple of many cyclists' diets, have a GI as high as 110, depending on variety (anything over 55 is considered high). And pasta can run into the 70s. Meanwhile, ice cream hovers around 30. What gives?

Fat and protein, that's what. Although ice cream is loaded with sugar, its fat and protein content slows the release of carbs into the bloodstream. But potatoes and pasta are very low in fat and protein, which means there's little to delay the dumping of sugar. This certainly doesn't mean you should stop eating pasta and potatoes. But the next time you eat either, note your reaction. Foods with a high GI tend to create sugar "highs" and subsequent lows, which can cause you to eat more than you actually need (this is also why diabetics are well-versed in the GI).

And there's yet another factor to consider: It's called glycemic load (if that nutritionist wasn't impressed by your grasp of the GI, blow them away with your understanding of GL). Glycemic load is determined by multiplying a food's GI by the grams of carbohydrate per serving. It's valuable information because some foods that are relatively high on the GI—carrots, for instance—actually carry a very low GL simply because they're not dense in calories. A normal or even abnormal serving of carrots isn't going to do much to your blood sugar levels because, with an average carrot running about 30 calories, you just can't eat enough to consume significant carbohydrates.

How does this fit into your nutritional plans? "Cyclists should emphasize low-GL foods in their day-to-day dietary habits," explains Dr. Applegate. "But during training and immediately following, it can be helpful to consume foods with a large GL because they'll have a more immediate impact on energy stores." Now you know.

Eating on the Bike

No matter how well you eat *off* the bike, you'll still need to eat *on* the bike, especially during rides that last more than 90 minutes. That's because exercise quickly depletes your stored muscle glycogen. Once that well starts to run dry, your cardiovascular system starts to depend more on blood glucose. To keep the pedals turning, you need to keep these sugar levels high.

Perhaps the most convenient way to do this is with an energy drink. There are literally dozens on the market, and all make some pretty outrageous claims. Your best bet is to experiment with a number of them during training (*never* during a race or an important event), to see which works best for you. Since most are formulated to fall in the 5 to 7 percent carbohydrate window that works best during exercise (check to be sure before you buy), consider mostly which one tastes best because you'll drink more frequently if you like the taste. And, of course, if any of them give you a bellyache, move on.

You can pretty much rely on an energy drink for rides up to 3 hours long. After that, you're going to want some solid food. There are numerous commercial energy bars and gels on the market; they're a fine, if expensive, way to keep you humming. Other good choices: bagels, bananas, and dried fruit, though everyone seems to have a favorite. Adventure mountain bike racer John Stamstead earned a dubious reputation for fueling with Spam and whole milk during races. I'm partial to chocolate chip cookies because I figure if I'm riding longer than 3 hours, a few chocolate chip cookies aren't going to hurt. If you're not using an energy drink for fuel, remember to hydrate with plain water.

A Matter of Fat

Next to carbohydrate, fat is your body's best fuel, especially on long, steady rides, when intensity is normally low. Still, this shouldn't be taken as license to eat all the ice cream and French fries you want (or even half as many as you want).

That's because while body fat is important for storing vitamins and providing insulation, most of us have plenty already. In fact, most of us have too much: While humans can store only limited amounts of glucose, the only limit on fat stockpiles is morbidity, which is not something you want to play around with.

Any kind of food can be stored as body fat (remember, it's excess calories that create body fat), but dietary fat is a common culprit. That's because it's present in many of the foods we most enjoy and because it contains more than twice as many calories per gram (9 per gram, rather than 4) as carbohydrate and protein.

Most nutritionists (at least those that haven't caught the Atkins bug) recommend that you derive no more than 30 percent of your total calories from fat and no more than 10 percent from the saturated fat found primarily in animal products. The remainder should be the unsaturated form that comes from vegetables oils, nuts, and grains.

One way to ensure a low fat intake is to check nutrition labels and select foods with fewer than 3 grams of fat per 100 calories. If this information is plainly listed, you can calculate the fat percentage this way: Look on the label for grams of fat per serving. Multiply this number by 9 (calories per gram of fat); then divide the result by the calories per serving. The result is the percentage of calories from fat. For example, one serving of a popular cheese spread has 80 calories and 6 grams of fat. So, 6 grams of fat × 9 calories per gram = 54 calories divided by 80 total calories = 67.5 percent of calories from fat. If you weren't already wondering what you were doing eating cheese spread instead of the real thing, this ought to make you think.

Still, let's be clear: Eating fat doesn't make you fat. Eating too much makes you fat. In fact, avoiding fat completely can cause you to eat *more* calories in the long run. That's because fat provides a feeling of satisfaction and fullness that carbohydrates—and, to a lesser extent, protein—can't. My personal experience suggests that you're better off eating a diet that feels right and not adding to your daily stress load by calculating every bite that goes into your body. I followed an extremely low fat diet for many years; at some point, I began adding more animal products, oils, nuts, and other "fatty" foods to my daily menus. I did not gain any weight, nor did my cholesterol rise. And I enjoying mealtimes a heck of a lot more!

Shedding Pounds

Cycling is an appealing weight-loss sport, because it's nonweight-bearing and burns gobs of calories. And because it's fun, it never seems like a burden.

If you've caught the cycling bug (and if you've read this far, consider yourself afflicted), you're halfway there: You've committed to exercise, which is absolutely critical to long-term weight loss.

The second commitment is harder: cutting calories. The bonus is that because of your commitment to riding, you needn't cut as nearly as many calories as a sedentary "dieter." In fact, unless your eating habits are seriously out of whack, your calorie cutting should be minimal enough that you'll hardly notice it. Remember: Cycling is a sport you can enjoy for the rest of your life, and for the rest of your life, it will help you manage your weight. Eat sensibly, ride lots, and enjoy both!

Power of Protein

Back in the good old days (say, about 5 years ago), protein-based diets were the stuff of bodybuilders and professional wrestlers. That's changed rapidly, with the advent of the Atkins (and Atkins-like) diet, which eschews carbohydrate in favor of protein and fat.

We've already discussed why these diets are not appropriate for a competitive cyclist. But we haven't talked about how much protein cyclists do need. Here's the short answer: Cyclists do need more protein than sedentary people. Of course, with every short, simple answer, there's a caveat, and here it is: Unless you adhere to a strict vegan diet that excludes animal products, you're probably already getting more than you need.

One reason cyclists need extra protein is for fuel. Yes, carbohydrate is the primary and preferred fuel for working muscles, but once it's been depleted, protein is pressed into service. "Protein can be a small but significant source of energy—about 5 to 10 percent of total energy needs," says researcher Michael J. Zackin, Ph.D., of the University of Massachusetts Medical School in Worcester. "Protein calories become increasingly important in carbohydrate-depleted states. If you train more than an hour a day and begin to deplete glycogen stores, you become increasingly dependent on body protein for energy."

Although results vary widely, Dr. Zackin says cycling may raise your protein requirements 20 to 90 percent beyond the U.S. recommended dietary allowance (RDA). The RDA is 0.363 gram of protein per pound of body weight. For a 150-pound person, this is about 54 grams per day. Add the 20 to 90 percent, and the 150-pound cyclist's daily protein need rises to between 65 and 103 grams.

That may seem like a lot, but most active people are already at these levels or beyond. This was illustrated in a study of eight highly trained female cyclists. Though their diets fell short of recommended values for several nutrients, their average protein intake was 145 percent of RDA. That's because high protein levels simply aren't hard to attain. For instance, 3 ounces of meat, fish, or poultry contains 21 grams of protein. A cup of beans has 14 grams; 3 tablespoons of peanut butter has 12; and a cup of fat-free milk contains 9. All of this adds up rather quickly. In fact, the average American consumes 100 grams of protein daily.

Instead of worrying about increasing your protein intake, consider where your protein comes from. The best sources are low in saturated fat and include a healthy dose of complex carbohydrates. Muscles are built by working them, not by feeding excessive protein, and the best fuel for work is (I'll say it one more time) complex carbohydrate. If you're eating an overall healthy diet that's rich in whole grains, beans, vegetables, fish, skinless poultry, soy products, lean meat, and nonfat dairy, you're getting plenty of protein. Vegetarians should fill their plates with grains, legumes, nuts, seeds, dairy products, and eggs. Vegans would be wise to consult a nutritionist to ensure they're getting adequate protein.

Supplementation

This is one of the more contentious issues in athletics. Does vitamin and mineral supplementation increase health and performance or just make expensive urine? The answer, to both questions, is a definite "yes."

Fact is, if you're eating a well-balanced diet, you're almost certainly getting all the vitamins and minerals you need. In fact, no research has found that taking supplements improves performance in adequately nourished cyclists. And some substances can actually accumulate to dangerous levels in your body if taken in large quantities. Too much niacin, for example, can cause rashes, nausea, and diarrhea, none of which will improve your cycling or any other facet of your life.

Of course, the other fact is it's almost impossible to always eat a well-balanced diet. And in truth, it's pretty difficult to overdose on vitamins, assuming you eat a normal diet and follow the manufacturer's suggested intake. So don't be scared of supplementation. If your schedule forces you to compromise on meals and has you running ragged, don't expect a supplement to set things straight. But it certainly won't hurt and can be viewed as relatively cheap insurance.

The Little Picture

If you're like most endurance athletes who've been blessed with neither pro contract nor lotto jackpot, your schedule demands some tough choices. And often those choices mean assuaging an empty belly with a pre-run energy bar or slurping a Cup-a-Soup on your way to the group ride. The problem? Powders, bars, supplements, and—surprise!—even pasta do not a performance diet make.

"Athletes are definitely going to a more refined diet, eating more processed and packaged foods," says Dr. Applegate. "They're saying 'Oh, well, this energy bar is fortified, so why can't I just live on these?'"

Consider the case of Adam Hodges Myerson, who began racing his road bike pretty seriously at age 15 around his hometown of Northampton, Massachusetts. Myerson racked up impressive results in short order; victories at the 1990 Fitchburg Stage Race and against the pros at that season's Marblehead road race had people nodding among themselves and saying "Hmm."

But Myerson knew little about nutrition; nor did he have the time to learn. His parents had recently divorced, and he found himself cooking for his three younger sisters, racing weekends, and navigating the turmoil of the separation. And as an ethical vegetarian, the challenge of procuring meat-free sustenance while traveling to races further muddied the water.

The result was a membership to what he now calls the Clif Bar culture. "I was subsisting on energy bars and peanut butter and Minute Rice and ramen," says Myerson, whose athletic coming of age coincided with the advent of commercial energy bars. "The teams I rode for were always sponsored by some bar or drink, so that stuff was always around."

And so were the lingering colds and other illnesses that caused Myerson to miss weeks of training each season. He was advised by more experienced racers to abandon his vegetarianism on the belief that such a diet could not sustain the day-in, day-out training loads of an elite cyclist. Myerson was convinced that the advice was misguided; he knew plenty of meat eaters who suffered the same symptoms. So Myerson examined his diet for other deficiencies and was startled at the volume of wrappers, jars, and boxes he'd left in his wake. He'd been competing on a diet almost entirely bereft of fruits, vegetables, grains, and legumes in their natural, unrefined state.

"Whole foods, and fruits and vegetables in particular, are packed with literally thousands of substances that protect them from the world they live in, things like ultraviolet light and bacteria in the soil," explains Dr. Applegate. "And guess what? The world they live in is the same one we live in." Chief among these substances are the phytochemicals that counteract the oxidative damage all exercise inflicts. It's oxidative damage that researchers believe can lead to cancer. Or a heart attack. Or any one of the dozens of chronic diseases you'd rather not harbor. More immediately, it's oxidative damage that makes you sore—and keeps you on the couch—the day after a hard workout. By bolstering your diet with foods rich in phytochemicals, you can drastically shorten the time it takes to recover from hard workouts. And, as we all know by now, the faster and more completely you recover, the sooner you can return to your training regimen.

Okay, sure, but you're getting your three or four servings a day, so what's to worry? Can a few energy bars really be that bad? No, they can't. But getting only three or four servings of whole food fruits and vegetables can be. In fact, the USDA has long recommended that active males looking to minimize their odds of contracting one of the previously mentioned diseases eat nine servings of fruits and veggies daily. Currently, barely 20 percent of Americans eat even five servings a day, according to a 2001 study commissioned by Produce For Better Health Foundation, a nonprofit organization based in Wilmington, Delaware, that champions the slaughter of millions of innocent snap peas. And nine servings? Try a piddling 2 percent of males ages 13 to 74.

This seems especially pathetic when one pauses to consider how easy it is to get those nine servings. Banana on your oatmeal and a glass of OJ—boom, there's two. Celery sticks and peanut butter midmorning. Tomato on your sandwich and a side salad at lunch—hey, you're up to five. At this rate, you'll hit double digits by the time you polish off your apple pie dessert (yeah, it counts; just go easy on the ice cream).

The core of Produce For Better Health's campaign is the tagline "Five a Day the Color Way." Its grade-school-ish rhyming scheme can be forgiven only because it so succinctly delivers the message: A healthy diet includes daily doses of five differently colored fruits and vegetables.

The key to that statement is the word "differently." That because of something called food synergy, which occurs only when foods are eaten in combination. Produce For Better Health's Christine Filardo, a registered dietitian, explains it this way: "Every nutrient has a certain action, but sometimes only when it's combined with other nutrients. It's a case of two plus two equaling more than four." In other words, an ear of corn and a tomato salad are more beneficial than two ears of corn.

Triathlete legend Dave Scott has been a whole-foods advocate since 1979, when preparations for the 1980 Ironman, combined with a refined-foods diet (he once consumed an 8½-pound ice cream sundae in one sitting), brought him to his knees. He concurs: "Every day there are more compounds identified in fruits and vegetables and grains. We don't really know how they work synergistically, but we know they do. Still, we're going the other way. People just get overwhelmed, say 'Screw that,' and start popping pills."

There's yet another problem with processed food that's inverse to why many athletes eat so much of it in the first place: control. Scott sees many of the professional and amateur athletes he coaches gravitating toward packaged food that's not just nonbeneficial but downright detrimental. "When you're working out 3 hours a day, it's so easy to rationalize and eat crappy food," he says. "But so much of that stuff is loaded with hydrogenated fat. One of the beauties of whole foods is that they just don't have that stuff."

Nor are they as calorically dense. Consider your average slice of cheesecake, which is dressed to kill in 300 calories. To get that sort of load out of, say, oranges, you'd have to eat five. First problem: You'd puke. Second problem: You're probably not going to stop at one piece of cheesecake. The blood sugar rush—and subsequent crash—will have you eyeing slice number two before you've even loosened your belt to accommodate the first.

All this is not to say endurance athletes (or anyone else, for that matter) need banish thoughtfully selected refined foods from their diet. Energy bars, sports powders, and well-chosen performance potions can—and probably should—find a place in your large intestine. "Energy foods are a wonderful invention," says Dr. Applegate. "They're convenient, and they give you exactly what you need when you're exercising. They just don't give you what you need to live on." Even Filardo allows that the convenience of these products often outweighs their nutritional deficiencies. "I'm not saying that you should never eat an energy bar. Sometimes it's the right thing. Before you do, though, think about this: How hard is it to instead grab an apple and a handful of nuts?" But if it means choosing between a Big Mac Value Meal and a couple of Clif Bars, well, it's not hard to figure out that you'd do better to give the golden arches wide berth.

And what of Adam Hodges Myerson, our bike-racing whole-foods convert? Rather than gnaw through a couple of bars in the hours before a workout or race, he now eats oatmeal topped with raisins, peanut butter, and soymilk. For recovery, he mixes his own smoothies with soymilk, frozen blueberries, bananas, and strawberries. The result? Myerson rarely misses a day of training due to illness, and his racing results have improved drastically.

7

ENDURANCE

Relevant to: All cycling disciplines

Endurance, loosely defined as the ability to ride for long periods, is the foundation for cycling fitness. Without adequate endurance, your body simply won't be able to keep going, no matter how much you feed it or swear at it.

Of course, different cycling disciplines require differing levels of endurance. Criterium races rarely last longer than an hour, while elite-level road races can last upwards of 6. If your goal is simply to be competitive in your chosen discipline, you need only develop the endurance necessary to finish your events strongly (though having greater endurance is almost never a liability).

Because building endurance doesn't demand high intensities, many people falsely assume it's the easiest facet of fitness to achieve. But it's actually one of the most difficult, especially for cyclists with busy lives. That's because there's simply no shortcut to endurance: You need to spend lots and lots of hours in the saddle, and you need to do it repeatedly. Once you have a strong endurance base, top-end fitness comes relatively quickly. But you've got to pay your dues.

Tips on Building Endurance

Make the Commitment

Begin by committing to a specific goal. Simply saying "I want to be able to ride longer" isn't going to cut it. Instead, pick a date and a distance (if you can tie this into an actual event, you'll be that much more motivated) and write time on your calendar (in ink, not pencil!). Be realistic: If you've never ridden longer than an hour at a shot, you're not riding 80 miles this coming Saturday. Figure on adding about 10 percent to your long ride every week; when you reach 75 percent of your target, you're ready. One rule: Never calculate your rides on mileage; your body knows only how long it's been riding, not how far. And because terrain and weather can have such an effect on average speed, the 20 miles you rode yesterday might take half again as long as the 20 miles you're going to ride tomorrow.

Look for Opportunity

To make serious fitness gains, you're going to need to ride at least three times each week. And to build endurance, at least one of these rides should "go long." For most of us, the greatest obstacle to endurance is life; that is, all the things we need to get done before we can get on the bike for a long ride.

One of the best solutions is to use your bike for transportation. Maybe you can set the alarm and take the "scenic" route to work. Or maybe you can ride to dinner at the in-laws' and have your family meet you there. If you're having trouble fitting your long ride into daylight hours, buy a bike light and some reflective clothing. Riding at night or in the early morning will seem odd at first, but you'll soon grow to love the sensation of punching through the dark in your own little world of light. Just be sure to seek out roads that are relatively free of traffic.

Gradually Build Your Mileage

Use the 10 percent rule to reduce the chance of injury or overtraining. If your longest ride is currently 90 minutes, next week shoot for 100, and the week after that, 110. If you're shooting for a target event that's based on mileage, not time, keep track of your average speed so you'll know when you're ready. Remember, as long as you can comfortably ride three-quarters of the time or distance you're aiming for, you'll do just fine.

Mimic the Event

Riding over terrain that's similar to your goal event isn't mandatory, but it will certainly help. You'll be physically and psychologically ready for whatever the event dishes out. Also, if it's a group event you're training for, try to find a group to train with. Not only will this build your group riding skills; it will also help the hours pass more quickly.

Practice the "Silent Skills"

Long, easy rides provide the perfect opportunity to practice all the little things that can make a big difference. Make sure you can change a flat tire on the road. Practice putting on a rain jacket and eating (not at the same time!) while riding. The fewer surprises you have on the big day, the smoother it will go.

Pace Yourself

Remember, you needn't ride at high intensities to build endurance. The goal of your long ride is to push the boundaries of time and distance, not speed. At the beginning of your ride, think about what you're going to feel like at the end, and remember that going fast in the first few miles is not going to help your cause (and might even force you to cut the ride short). Pacing yourself is especially important when riding in a group, where the dynamics of competition can quickly force the pace beyond what you're comfortable with. Try to find a group with similar goals, and don't be afraid to drop off the back.

On the other hand, don't waste time. Dawdling at convenience stores or coffee shops doesn't build endurance, unless you're training for the espresso-drinking world championships. Stop just long enough to stock up on food and water, and then keep pedaling.

Tank Up

Food and fluid are absolutely critical for long rides. Since these rides are typically done at low intensities, you can eat a preride meal shortly before you leave. Bring enough food (or enough money to buy food, assuming there are smart food choices on your route) so that you can eat at least 300 calories for each hour on the bike (about half of what you'll burn), and plenty of water. How much water is plenty? That depends largely on weather conditions, but if you're not stopping to urinate at least once every 2 hours, you're not drinking enough.

Divide to Conquer

A long ride is as much a mental challenge as a physical feat. If 3 hours sounds daunting, consider: It's just three hour-long rides. Don't dwell on the big obstacles coming up; instead, enjoy the scenery and the feeling of wind and sun on your face (or, if it's raining, the feeling of water on your face).

If you begin to struggle, set short-term goals. Tell yourself that you'll take a pit stop at the next store, or at the top of the hill, or wherever make sense. Turn your macro goal into a series of micro goals that are easily attained. And if all else fails, think about what you're going to eat when you get home!

8

SPEED

Relevant to: criteriums, road racing, group rides
In cycle-speak, the word "speed" means more than simply riding fast. It's also a riding style, the ability to accelerate quickly, turning the pedals at a high rate and putting in a burst that leaves the competition reeling in your wake (hey, you might as well think big).

Many cyclists never perform specific speed training because they see no practical need for it. And while it's true that enthusiast cyclists rarely need to uncork a fearsome sprint, it's also true that everyone can

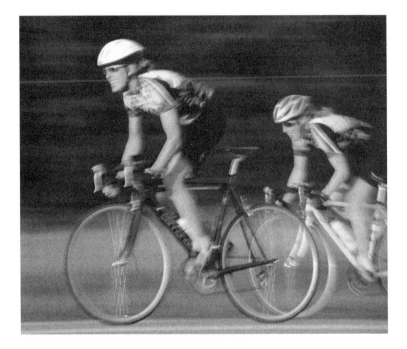

benefit from the ability. For instance, group rides often feature hotly contested "town line" sprints, in which riders sprint for the road signs that mark a town's border. True, there's no prize money involved, but the bragging rights that go along with winning a town line sprint are priceless. And consider what a well-developed sprint can do for you when a charging Doberman comes boiling out of its yard. In this situation, speed is definitely your friend (as is a can of pepper spray).

These situations demand the same skill as the charge to the finish line of a hotly contested road race or criterium: You must accelerate to high speed and hold that speed for a few seconds. It's a skill that goes to the very core of what's great about riding a bicycle, and it's one that's surprisingly easy to develop.

Speedwork

Conventional interval training helps you ride faster, but its main objectives are the development of aerobic and anaerobic capacity.

When you do intervals, each intense effort is followed by easier riding that allows only partial recovery, at which point you go hard again. Speedwork is different. The hard efforts are very hard; essentially, as hard as you can go. But they are (blessedly) brief and separated by enough time for complete recovery. For instance, as little as 10 seconds of all-out effort may be followed by as much as 5 minutes of easy spinning. The emphasis is on acceleration and leg speed, not heart rate (in fact, due to a phenomenon known as heart-rate lag, you won't even see a very high heart rate during your sprint—though it'll likely keep climbing in the first seconds of your recovery period).

Speedwork isn't actually very taxing, and can be implemented into any otherwise easy ride, as often as twice each week. Just be sure to warm up for at least 15 minutes first; then do five to eight sprints of 10 to 30 seconds each, with full recovery in between. Use gears that you won't completely spin out, and really concentrate on the elements of good technique described on page 43. Remember, you're training your pedaling style and speed, as much as your fitness.

This whole workout takes less than an hour (though you can easily sandwich it into a longer ride; in fact, this is what many pro riders do). After several weeks, you'll notice improvement in your top-end speed and acceleration. Perhaps more importantly, so will your competition.

Spin City

Conventional wisdom says that speed can be raised in two ways: by increasing cadence (pedaling faster) or by increasing power (pedaling harder) so you can use a bigger gear at a given cadence. Conventional wisdom isn't wrong (it rarely is), but there's a third key to quickness that is often neglected: technique. Without efficient form, a cycling with the speed of a cheetah and the power of a Mack truck will waste much of it on flailing legs, flying elbows, and bobbing shoulders. Speed depends on cadence and technique, so let's talk about how to improve them.

The simplest way to cultivate fast, smooth leg speed is to spin low-to-moderate gears at high rpm. In fact, you should work on this before beginning formal speedwork. If your normal cruising cadence is around 90 rpm, start there and gradually increase it to 100, 110, even 120, until your legs lose coordination and you're bouncing in the saddle like a jumping bean. At this point, ease back a few rpm and hold it there for a few seconds; then inch it up again. Repeat this sequence several times. After a few sessions, your maximum cadence and the fastest smooth cadence you can sustain will both rise. (Big bonus: this is going to make you look soooo much smoother—and therefore pro—on your bike)

Use gradual downhills to help get your leg speed up without undue cardiovascular stress (from an aerobic standpoint, these workouts should be easy to moderate). Instead of shifting into a bigger gear as you descend, stay in lower gears and let gravity help turn your legs into a blender. You can also use a tailwind to the same effect, though who among us can resist shifting up a few gears and using Ma Nature's helping hand to hit crazy speeds?

Once you're comfortable with this exercise, move on to low-gear intervals. Instead of using big gears or climbs at 80 to 90 rpm to develop power and increase your anaerobic threshold, use small gears and a high cadence (110 to 120 rpm). One-minute intervals done in this fashion will continue to improve coordination as they condition your cardiovascular system and fast-twitch muscles, two key ingredients of a killer sprint. Because it puts minimal strain on tendons and joints, this workout is fantastic for early in the season, while your body is still adapting to the bike.

When you start doing these exercises, your pedal stroke is bound to feel choppier than a Cuisinart. Focus on relaxing your entire body. Keep your shoulders and arms loose and quiet by holding the handlebar only as tight as you need to maintain control. Try to confine all motion to your legs, which will help keep your hips from bouncing. Encourage smoothness by goading yourself to pedal faster, not harder. This approach works anytime you want to turn the pedals quicker, no matter what gear you're in.

Technique Tips

There are three major technique flaws most riders commit when they're sprinting out of the saddle. By avoiding these, you will greatly improve your ability to accelerate and hold your speed, even with no increase in fitness (you're not going to hear that often, so enjoy it).

1. Riders tend to move their upper bodies too much. Your back should act like a fulcrum, and shouldn't move. When your upper body is kept still, it serves as a brace for the power of your legs. Your arms should move only enough to let the bike sway from side to side in rhythm with your pedal strokes.

2. Cyclists tend to move their weight too far forward. When you stand to spring, your shoulders should be only as far forward as the front axle. Lean forward more than that, and you'll encounter several speed-sapping problems. You'll have too much weight on your front wheel, which will make the bike unstable and hard to handle. Your hips will be too far forward in relation to the crankset, which means you won't be able to get as much leverage on the pedals. And your head will be down, making it difficult to see where you're going—not good when you're sprinting at maximum speed.

3. Cyclists use their upper body incorrectly. When sprinting, you should pull on the handle bar with a rowing motion to balance the power in your legs. If you don't, the bike will be more apt to flop from side to side, wasting power and control, something no one can afford to lose.

9

FORCE

Relevant to: All cycling disciplines

Force is simple to understand: "If you want to ride hard," says cycling coach Joe Friel, author of *The Cyclist's Training Bible*, "you need to be able to push down on the pedals real hard." That, in plain terms, is force, and it's a crucial building block of cycling fitness.

There are numerous ways to develop force, but the most popular are weight lifting, hill training, and pushing big gears. None of these are without risk (mostly for injury), but as Friel puts it, "cycling is like investing in stocks: The higher the risk, the higher the potential reward." The key is to implement force thoughtfully and carefully, and only after you've cultivated a solid base.

To make your pedaling more forceful, be prepared to hurt. A lot. Although on-the-bike force-building efforts are generally conducted at lower intensities than power intervals, they last a lot longer and take serious mental fortitude to get through. But it's important to grin and bear it because gaining force is like opening a door into a new world of cycling fitness.

Force Training

Force intervals are long efforts that are conducted at or slightly above your anaerobic threshold. Basically, you're going to go as hard as you possibly can for the prescribed duration, which should start at about 3 minutes and increase by approximately 1 minute each workout. You should use a gear that demands a slightly lower cadence than normal; if 90 rpm is normal for you, shoot for about 80 rpm during these efforts. You're going to start with a total of 9 minutes of intervals and gradually build to twice that. These intervals are best done on flat surfaces or low-grade climbs.

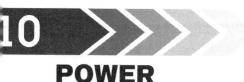

POWER

Relevant to: All cycling disciplines, but especially climbing, time trialing, and mountain biking

Earlier, we talked a bit about training with power meters and about the importance of maximizing your power-to-weight ratio. But we didn't talk much about how to actually increase power, whether you're using a meter or not. Here's where we get down to it.

Power has a precise meaning to physiologists. It's defined as force multiplied by velocity, and physics says that the power required to overcome air drag is proportional to the cube of the velocity.

"Oh, great," you're thinking. "Now I have to carry a calculator on all my rides." Don't fret: All you need to know about power is that you want it. It's what gets you over steep climbs without resorting to the humiliation of your granny gear, and it's what helps you hold an impressive pace in the face of a tough headwind. In its most base, cycle-friendly terms, power is the ability to keep the crankarms turning when the resistance rises.

Sounds great, huh? It is. But like so many great things, it doesn't come easily. And you need gobs of it to make a dramatic difference. In fact, thanks to wind resistance (remember all that chatter about overcoming air drag being proportional to the cube of the velocity?), if you want to increase your speed from 20 to 25 mph, you need to double your power. Umph. What's that, you say? You want to double your speed from, say, 15 to 30 mph? No problem. A mere eightfold increase in power will do it (all other factors being equal). Consider now-retired English pro Chris Boardman, who set a world record by riding more than 34 miles in a single hour around an indoor velodrome. Now, that's *power*.

Power lets you ride more explosively, too. With power, you can sprint in a bigger gear, which lets you cover ground faster. You know you need to work on power when you encounter these situations: You can't sprint in a gear that's big enough to make you competitive; you can't maintain the group's speed when you reach the front of the paceline; you have trouble getting back into the paceline after taking your pull; you find it impossible to accelerate during a climb; headwinds force you into low gears; and rides that require frequent pace changes leave you overly tired.

There's little doubt that one, two, or even more of these will ring a bell with you. Don't be discouraged: They're ringing a bell with everyone that is reading this book. That's because power is the single most important factor in a cyclist's fitness. And, in a classic case of Murphy's Law, the single hardest thing to earn.

Power Training

Working on power means sometimes riding with a relatively low cadence, in a relatively large gear (for this reason, you should begin power work only after you've developed a strong base of miles). Instead of the leg-blurring spin of speedwork sprints, you may find yourself chugging along at 70 rpm—or even lower. This is especially true on hills, where you'll intentionally remain in gears that force you to drive the pedals, rather than shift lower and spin as you would during a typical ride.

There are a wide variety of ways to develop power. One is with hard accelerations in a big gear. For instance, roll along at 40 rpm in a large gear, stay seated, and accelerate as hard as you can for 10 to 30 seconds. Recover by spinning a much lower gear, and repeat the cycle five to eight times. You can accomplish much the same thing by riding in rolling terrain and charging up short hills in the saddle without shifting down or letting your cadence drop (in fact, you should try to increase it). On longer climbs, stay seated as long as possible, and then, just as you start to fade, stand and shift into a harder gear. Or repeatedly slow and then accelerate all the way up. If there is a dearth of long climbs where you ride, use headwinds to your advantage: Select a moderately big gear and keep your cadence at a steady 75 rpm as you climb the "invisible hill."

Sounds like a blast, eh? Well, it's not easy to develop the cardio-vascular fitness, muscle strength, and energy systems that power demands. Much of this work will occur at or above your lactate threshold. This means two things: You're going to suffer. And you need to be careful. This is just the sort of riding that can spiraling into the abyss of overtraining. Too, it puts a lot of strain on delicate tendons and ligaments. Start with just one power training session per week, and never do more than two.

Note: Because these are such short efforts, a heart-rate monitor is practically useless. Instead, ride off of perceived exertion which, in this case, is pretty simple, if painful: Go as hard as you absolutely freakin' can.

Recovering from Force and Power Training

For best gains, and to help avoid overtraining, be sure to plan easy recovery rides for the days before and after a force or power workout. In fact, you may want to take two easy days after a particularly demanding ride. A common training program calls for Monday rest after a hard weekend of riding and racing, speedwork on Tuesday, steady endurance riding on Wednesday, force or power work on Thursday, and an easy spin for recovery on Friday. Of course, this schedule is sweeping in its generalization, but with some tweaking to fit your personal goals and lifestyle, it's a good place to start.

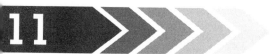

BRAIN TRAINING

Danish cycling coach and winner of the 1996 Tour de France Bjarne Riis has earned a reputation as a man who can take good riders and make them great. Perhaps the best example of this is Ivan

Basso, who had a reputation of his own: talented rider, but too nice and mild-mannered to be a true winner.

Riis didn't believe it and lured Basso away from his support rider position on the Italian Fassa Bortolo team late in 2003. Basso signed with Riis's CSC squad as a team leader and began preparations to take on the 2004 Tour de France, the world's largest bicycle race, with an eye on the podium.

The skeptics thought that Basso couldn't do it, that he lacked the killer instinct and unrelenting drive it took to contend a major 3-week bicycle race. But Riis knew better, and when Basso took to the roads of France, he was a rider transformed. He rode with utter confidence, marking Lance Armstrong in the high mountain terrain and riding consistently throughout the 3-week race, eventually finishing third.

Confidence breeds confidence, so perhaps it's no surprise that in 2005, Basso upped his game again, contesting both the Tour and the Giro d'Italia, the world's second-hardest bike race. Few modern riders compete in both events; it's simply considered too difficult, but Basso turned in stunning performances. Only a punk stomach kept him from winning the Giro, and in the Tour, he again rode with quiet confidence to finish second. Even Armstrong was impressed: At the podium presentation in Paris, he went so far as to tip Basso as the 2006 winner.

The transformation was complete. Ivan Basso had become a true champion, a legendary cyclist whose name will remain in the record books for all of cycling history. How did Riis do it? How did he take a good rider and turn him into a truly great rider? As Basso himself has said, it's simple: He believed in his rider.

Most people understand the value of tools such as wrenches and screwdrivers: They help keep bikes running well. Like these tools, most of the techniques discussed in this book are easy to grasp and quickly useful. Others, though, are a little harder to get a handle on. One of the most intangible is confidence. Ivan Basso always had the talent; what he lacked was the confidence to make the most of it. Without that confidence, he was condemned to ride below his true potential.

Sounds good, but how do you gain confidence, especially with limited experience?

The first key is focus. To be a successful cyclist, you need to set goals, whether it's gearing up for a century ride or big race, or just trying to get over the next hill. By focusing on these goals, you lay the foundation for confidence because nothing inspires confidence like knowing you've specifically prepared and ready to attain your goals.

Focus can be described as narrowed attention. Focus is concentration. It lets you aim your vision and define your view. You choose a distant goal (usually a major event or ride) and commit to preparing for it. Staying focused on the goal—sustaining a strong mental image of the event—makes it easier to put in the necessary work. It will get you out the door on rides you might otherwise be tempted to skip, rides that, once completed, build confidence.

Zeroing In

Short-term focus is the ability to clear your mind of everything extraneous and concentrate on the task at hand. For example, working on your sprint for the race in 2 weeks instead of obsessing about the district championship in 6 weeks, or finishing the last 5 miles of today's 60-mile training race instead of fretting about the century in 2 months.

Successful short-term focus also means that at crucial moments you think only about cycling. For most busy adults, that may seem like a tall order, but try to remember that dwelling on the other responsibilities in your life while you're on the bike isn't going to make them go away.

Imagine yourself riding in a group at a brisk pace, your front wheel a mere whisper away from the rear wheel of the rider in front of you. Every rider must keep a uniform speed and ride a straight line, lest the entire group come tumbling down. This is no time to have your mind on the argument you just had with your spouse, or the latest crisis at work. In the most intense moments in cycling, as in life, the likelihood of making a mistake increases if you don't have complete focus. You may not even notice that your mind wanders at crucial times. On your next few rides, pay attention to how your mental state relates to various situations, and consider if it's a hindrance or a help.

Studies have compared endurance athletes who zero in with those who zone out during events. Riders who focus on the task at hand (zero in) perform better. This is called association. The opposite, disassociation, is less productive because you take yourself out of the task rather than commit to it. The next time you see Lance Armstrong or Tyler Hamilton flying up a climb, take a look at his expression. What do you see? Supreme focus. Association.

This isn't to say you must concentrate solely on cycling for every minute of every ride. It's natural to let your mind wander, and even beneficial in certain circumstances. But particularly during hard efforts and races, focused concentration is a key component to performance.

The Grin Factor

If you're thinking that all this means a grim-faced take on cycling, think again because focus can actually make your riding more fun. That's because, quite simply, focus, and the confidence that results, brings about better riding. Think about ripping down a technical singletrack descent. Sounds like a blast, right? But to make it down without kissing a tree or some dirt, you're going to need supreme focus. Focus makes you faster. Focus makes it fun.

So there you have it. The fundamentals. Endurance. Power. Speed. Focus. With these four ingredients, you can mix a potent cocktail of cycling fitness that will take your riding to new levels.

12

THE SUBJECTIVE CYCLIST

Too often, discussions of training technique and theory conveniently ignore one simple fact: At even a professional level, riding your bike is only a small fraction of what you do on a day-in, day-out basis. Even if you ride an average of 3 hours a day, 7 days a week, that's "only" 21 hours on your bike out of 168 total hours in the week. The point is that those other 147 hours have a tremendous impact on your training and the results of your training. That's because your central nervous system can withstand only so much stress, whether that stress comes as a result of hard training, or an argument with your significant other/boss/kids/parents.

"Emotion is a stress that can have tangible effects," says Rick Crawford, a cycling coach based in Durango, Colorado. "Stress can come from pushing a wheelbarrow all day, riding your bike, or worrying about your finances. The problem is you can't put a power meter on a fight with your spouse. How do you quantify it? You can't, really. But there's no doubt it has an impact on an athletes."

Crawford uses the convenient analogy of a wheel, with the central nervous system (CNS) acting as the hub, and the spokes playing the role of the varying facets of life. "The CNS defines the entire physical and spiritual composition of the rider, the emotions, nervous tissue, heart, and soul of the athlete," explains Crawford.

Consider the case of Tom Danielson. Four years ago, Danielson was a talented but struggling mountain bike racer at Fort Lewis College in Durango. Crawford, the team's coach, had tested Danielson and knew the kid had phenomenal talent. But the talent was buried under a heaping pile of life stress. "I was just a stress case," remembers Danielson, who joined Lance Armstrong's Discovery Channel team in 2004. "I was strong, but couldn't function properly. At first, I didn't really understand how it was affecting my riding. I was like 'What do you mean? I should train less because I've having trouble with my girlfriend?' But you know what? It made all the difference in the world."

Indeed. Once Danielson started acknowledging life stress and factoring it into his training program, his results skyrocketed. He won the collegiate mountain bike nationals and launched a road racing career that many expect will eventually culminate in a Tour de France win.

According to Crawford, you can't compartmentalize training and life stress, which is why he likes the wheel analogy: Just like a real bicycle wheel, it takes only one broken spoke to throw the whole thing out of whack. And what are those spokes? There might be one for work stress, another for family, and yet another for financial worries. Then there's sleep quality, diet, and training. And so on. Just about anything you think about or do can be a spoke that affects the integrity of your "life wheel."

Lest you think this is something only professional riders need worry about, think again: "This is especially true for an amateur rider, who has a family and 9-to-5 job," says Crawford. "Professionals have the luxury of living in a vacuum, where training and racing are the priorities. Not many of us can do that."

So how do you determine if your languid legs are the result of too little training or too much life stress? Although there's no definitive measurement tool, Crawford has developed a formula that can help pinpoint the cause. It's called Stress Score, and here's how it works. In a notebook, rank your physical, mental, and emotional tolls on a scale of 1 to 10 (10 being the highest stress level). For instance, you might be suffering from a cold or recovering from a hard day of training, which would put your physical score at, say, a 9. If things are going smoothly at work and home, your mental score might be relatively low, say 3. But maybe you're a bit depressed about being sick and you're having a hard time motivating to do things that you're normally excited about, so your emotional mark will be an 8. The total is 20, and this is your Debit Score.

Next, consider a variety of credit factors, which Crawford lists as sleep, rest (what you're doing when you're not sleeping), and therapy (anything that helps you cope with life stress). So, if you slept well the night before, you'd get a high score there. And if the physical demands on your day are light, you'd get another high mark. Next, consider your outlets for coping for the debit side of the equation. Are they in place? Are they accessible? Again, rate the access and effectiveness of this "therapy." Total up these three numbers to get your Credit Score.

"It's no different than balancing a checkbook," says Crawford, who suggests carrying a running Stress Score, just as you would carry a running balance in your checkbook. Every 3 weeks, says Crawford, you should zero out your Stress Score by, in essence, pampering yourself. "It might take a week; it might take 2 weeks," says Crawford. "But you won't believe the difference it will make."

This may be hard medicine to swallow because often the only stress that's flexible in a busy cyclist's life is their training schedule. But according to Crawford, an undertrained cyclist with a fresh CNS is better off than a well-trained rider whose CNS is on the brink of collapse. "To take advantage of your fitness, you need a CNS that can generate spark," he explains. "For most riders, being excited is more important than that last few percent of fit." Another benefit is longevity: By monitoring and correcting your stress levels, you're much less likely to burn out after only a season or two. Or, as Crawford says, "Ninety-eight percent for 10 years is better than 200 percent for 1 year."

Over the long term, keep an eye on what generates stress in your life. "You can't believe the revelatory powers of this system," says Crawford. "It's a life changer. Suddenly, you're accounting for your life."

13 >>>>

TESTING

How do you know if a training program is working for you? Most riders rely on a combination of race performances and riding sensations to monitor the effectiveness of their programs. And while those are very important guidelines, it's also important to implement a repeatable test, especially if your competitions are few and far between.

There are multitude ways to do this. Top athletes often use expensive laboratory equipment to measure sophisticated fitness markers such as lactic acid levels and max VO_2. You, presumably, do not have the access or the sponsor backing to make regular lab testing part of your program. But that doesn't mean you can't accurately test your progress (or lack thereof). In fact, real-world field tests hold significant advantages over contrived laboratory testing. They're free, for one. For another, they're easy to repeat, allowing you to test your progress regularly. (But not frequently: This is a hard effort that should count as one of your hard training days. You'll repeat this test every 6 weeks throughout the season). And finally, you don't ride and race in a lab, so whatever parameters you establish there do not directly correlate to the real world passing beneath your wheels.

To create your baseline test, choose a section of road that takes about 10 minutes to ride at a hard pace. It needn't be a specific distance or take a specific amount of time to complete (10 minutes is about right, but you could go a few minutes below or above that), but it should have definite and easily identifiable beginning and end points. It should *not* be off-road because weather conditions will have a far greater impact on the terrain (and thus the amount of time it takes you to complete the test) than they do on paved roads. Flat or rolling terrain is preferable, and make sure to mark out a section of road that's free of stop signs and lights and is relatively free of traffic. You want as few distractions as possible.

Once you've selected the appropriate slice of road, you're ready. Make sure you're well-rested, hydrated, and warmed up before tackling your test course. In other words, approach your baseline testing as you would any hard ride or race. You're going to ask a lot of your body; you need to give it every opportunity to perform to its maximum.

Also make sure you're equipped to record the following:

- Time of day (try to keep this consistent across all tests throughout the season)
- Duration of effort (assuming you're riding a set distance)
- Distance of effort (if you're riding for a set time)
- Average heart rate

- Average power (if you have a power meter, obviously)

- Weather conditions

- Perceived effort (how you felt, regardless of what the numbers say)

- Other factors (this could be anything you felt contributed to or detracted from your performance)

Once you've warmed up for at least 15 minutes (including a couple of short, 1- or 2-minute high-intensity efforts to "wake up" your body and mind), arrive at the "start line" of your test course. Choose a gear that allows you to get into a comfortable, high cadence quickly and settle into the effort. Remember that you're going to be riding very hard for about 10 minutes, and try to pace yourself accordingly. Likewise, if you're not suffering, you're not going hard enough. This should hurt, just not so much that you can't maintain it for the full distance.

This is a good opportunity to experiment with different cadences. Once you're up to speed, try shifting gears while maintaining the same rate. Note how your heart rate reacts. If it drops a beat or two at a certain cadence with no change in pace, you've just found some free speed. Cherish it because it doesn't come around too often.

At the completion of your baseline test, you should feel as if you couldn't have ridden any faster for that distance. Record your numbers, and spin home easily to cool down and reflect on the effort. If you think you could have gone harder, remember that feeling and save it for your next test.

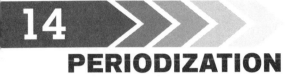

PERIODIZATION

This fancy, made-up word is based on a simple concept: No athlete can be 100 percent ready all the time. Indeed, few amateur cyclists are capable of maintaining a race-winning level of fitness for more than 3 or 4 weeks at a time before their bodies and minds begin to wilt under the stress.

The failure to embrace this reality is what leads many athletes down a dead-end road to burnout. Think of your body as a high-performance car: If you go around revving the engine to redline all the time, it's not going to last very long. But if you take care of it, pamper it with good fuel and proper rest, it will be ready to run hard when you need it to.

The idea, then, is to deconstruct your season with a focus on the events—be they races, club centuries, or charity rides—that are most important to you. You should do this well in advance of the season, as soon as you can confirm the scheduling of key events. January is not too early, though if you're targeting only a single event that's later in the season, you have a bit more flexibility. But you should develop your plan at least 3 months before your priority event.

The best way to do this is to buy a calendar and jot down all the events that you want to do. Then flip back through the months and put a star or check mark next to events that are particularly important to you—the events you want to complete at peak fitness. Now run through your calendar again and note where these priority events fall in relation to each other.

Here's where things get tricky. Remember, you're not going to be able to hold on to peak fitness for more than a few weeks (if you're new to structured training, it's probably more like 10 days). That's the bad news. The good news is you can reach this fitness peak more than once in a season. In fact, depending on how long your season and how long you try to maintain top fitness, you can peak as many as three times over the cycling season. That's because it takes 9 to 12 weeks to recover from one peak and build to the next. Look at your priority events again. How many are there? How far apart are they? To reach peak fitness for each, they'll need to be spread far enough apart to allow you to recover from the previous fitness peak and build toward the next one. Conversely, you might also cluster two priority events and complete both during the same fitness peak. The point is, you simply cannot expect to be 100 percent for every event on your calendar. In fact, to be 100 percent for any of them means being much less than 100 percent at most of them, unless you're targeting only two or three events.

Let's say you have four priority events on your calendar. The dates are June 3, June 24, September 1, and September 8. Right away, you have a hard choice to make because the June events are too far apart to maintain a peak and not far enough apart to target separately. Your best bet is to focus on the June 24 event, which will allow you to use the June 3 event as "practice." Top professionals have long used competition as "practice": Lance Armstrong's domineering performances at the Tour de France were preceded by less dominant showings at smaller stage races. This is in many regards an ideal situation, so long as you're able to detach emotionally from your performance in the first event.

The key to making "practice" events work for you is being able to detach emotionally from your performance in the event. If you do poorly, you need to remember that you're not there for the glory; you're there to refine your racing strategies and skills, something that can be accomplished no matter where you finish. Or even if you finish.

The September events, on the other hand, are close enough together to tackle in the same peak. With careful attention to training (and this book!), you'll ride into September with a high level of fitness and storm through those events with more power and speed than you thought possible.

Grab your calendar again, and count back 12 weeks, which

should—no joke—land you on April 1. Make a big red X, a check mark, or a smiley face on March 1. Why? Because that's when your training must begin to get serious. (Bear in mind the word "begin." That's because the 3-month time frame assumes you're carrying some basic fitness into it. If all you're carrying is a winter's worth of pork rinds, you should take a longer view. But if you're serious enough to have read this far, it's fairly safe to assume you've kept somewhat active through the colder months.)

The Base Period

This does not mean that once March 1 rolls around, you're going to attack the pedals like never before. In fact, you'd do better instead to exercise restraint and focus your training energies on longer, easier rides. This is knows as the base period, and it's during this period that you'll start to develop the most basic components of cycling fitness: endurance, force, and speed.

It's also during this period that you'll actually increase your ability to endure harder training simply by going slow. Sounds like a neat trick, right? Well, it's not really a trick; it's a physiological fact that low-intensity riding encourages the development of oxygen-carrying capillaries in your muscles. And when the chips are down, your muscles want oxygen. Lots of it. Oxygen is like jet fuel, like a turbocharger, like . . . You get the point. And the more supply lines (capillaries), the more you can feed your muscles. But remember this: These capillaries are produced only during low-intensity riding. That's why you need to think of this period as an investment in your riding future. The more you invest now, the more you'll reap later.

In fact, you should spend the first 6 to 8 weeks of bike-specific training at low intensity (65 to 80 percent of your anaerobic threshold heart rate, ATHR). This is called "base training" because it is what every successful cycling season is built on. If you're champing at the bit to go harder, good. That's enthusiasm you can harness for later, when tough training and racing will demand all you've got and more. For now, remember that your goals are long-term and that the slower you go now, the faster you'll go later. (This is a good time of the year to avoid group rides, which can quickly turn into impromptu races, no matter what promises are made at the outset).

During this 6- to 8-week period, slowly ratchet up the duration and frequency of your rides, taking care not to exceed the previous week's total by more than 10 percent, expressed as time, not miles. For instance, if your 1st week of training yields 6 on-the-bike hours, with a long ride of 90 minutes, your 2nd week of training should total no more than 6½ hours, with a long ride of approximately 1:40. Build your 3rd week (7:15, long ride of 1:50) on your 2nd, but on the 4th week, ease off, riding only two-thirds of your 1st week's total (4:00). On week 5 (8:00, long ride of just over 2:00), build on the 3rd week's hours, and continue building for weeks 6 and 7. On week 8, drop back to week 1's training load.

Going into week 9, you can begin upping the pace by incorporating low-intensity muscular endurance (ME) intervals into your schedule. ME intervals are not all-out efforts; instead, they're designed to prepare your body for the truly hard training to come. Still, they're going to be much more challenging than anything you've done thus far. But if you're like most ambitious cyclists, the increase in pace will come as a relief after so many weeks of low-intensity riding.

You'll begin with two ME interval sessions per week. You can do these on whatever days you want, so long as you space them as far apart as possible. In other words, shoot for Wednesday and Sunday, or Thursday and Monday, or whatever works for your schedule.

For your very first session, shoot for 20 minutes of total interval time, divided into 4- or 5-minute intervals. The recovery between intervals should be fairly short, about 25 percent of the interval time. In other words, a 4-minute ME interval would be followed by 1 minute of easy spinning before you begin the next effort. These short recovery periods teach your body to recover quickly, which will help you withstand the frequent accelerations of racing. On every subsequent interval workout, add a minute to each interval, until they're 10 to 12 minutes each.

One crucial point: The numbers above should serve as a guideline only. Don't exceed them, and don't feel like you're cheating if you need to cut the session short. There's one little-known rule that will help you get the most out of your training: Always head home feeling as if you could have done one more interval. Too many athletes ride until utter exhaustion, heading home only when forced to because their tongue is caught in the spokes of their front wheel. By cutting your interval workouts just short of complete physical breakdown, you'll be able to recover much more quickly, which means a speedy return to quality training.

As mentioned, the intensity of these ME intervals is fairly low. "Most riders want to make these way too difficult," says Joe Friel, a top cycling coach and author of *Cyclist's Training Bible*. "You should be just starting to redline, never maxed out." That means you should shoot for a heart rate that's a beat or three below your anaerobic threshold. Finally, to help develop force, you should perform these intervals in a gear that forces you to maintain a cadence about 10 percent lower than normal. In other words, if your cadence typically runs about 90 rpm, select a gear that puts you at 80 rpm.

If you've never done intervals before, congrats. You've just completed a rite of passage that marks the transformation from recreational to serious cyclist. Stick with it, and great things are sure to come.

After 3 weeks of ME intervals, again schedule an easy, recovery week. This might be hard to do because you'll probably be seeing some big gains in fitness and force. But it's important because things are about to get a whole lot harder.

Turning Up the Heat

If you've timed things right, you're now 10 to 12 weeks from your first priority event, and it's time to begin the high-intensity training that will deliver you to the start iine with the fitness you need to be competitive.

Even with a solid base of low intensity and ME riding in your legs, it's critical to introduce high-intensity training slowly and thoughtfully. Remember, at no point should high-intensity training comprise more than 20 percent of total riding time. In fact, when it's first introduced, it should be much less, perhaps half that.

The next step is the introduction of high-intensity, anaerobic endurance (AE) intervals. AE intervals are performed just above your anaerobic threshold; these are the efforts that are really going to push the top end of your fitness, both by increasing your ability to perform at or above your AT and by actually raising your AT.

AE intervals are shorter than ME efforts for one simple reason: They're harder. While ME intervals happen just below your anaerobic

SAMPLE BASE WEEK »»»

Monday: OFF or short, easy ride below 80% ATHR

Total Duration: 60 minutes

Intensity: Low

Tuesday: Base ride

Total Duration: 60–120 minutes

Intensity: Low-medium (below 88% ATHR)

Wednesday: ME workout as described on previous pages (only after 8 weeks of base training; otherwise, base ride)

Total Duration: 60–90 minutes

Intensity: Medium-high

Thursday: Base ride

Total Duration: 60–120 minutes

Intensity: Low-medium

Friday: OFF

Saturday: Base ride

Total Duration: 90–180 minutes

Intensity: Low-medium

Sunday: ME workout or base ride

Total Duration: 60–90 minutes

Intensity: Medium-high

Total Hours: **6.5–11**

threshold, your AE efforts will be at 3 to 10 beats above your AT. This, friends, is the pain zone. Fortunately, you needn't spend a lot of time there. Your first set of AE intervals should consist of five 3-minute efforts, for a total of 15 minutes of interval time. The recovery ratio for these is a bit more generous; you should take 3 minutes of easy spinning for every interval for a 1:1 recovery ratio. Again, you're going to perform this workout twice each week, and you should increase the length of your intervals at each workout by 30 seconds (also increase your recovery time to maintain the 1:1 ratio).

You should do two 3-week blocks of AE training, separated and followed by a recovery week of easy spinning at base-level intensities. By the end of this period, you should be seeing significant improvements in your ability to withstand and maintain high intensities. Loosely translated: You'll be dropping riding partners who only weeks ago left you in their wake.

A word of warning: With this type of high-intensity riding, you're tiptoeing on fairly thin ice in regard to overtraining. Keep a very close watch on overtraining symptoms, such as elevated resting heart rate, a decrease in appetite, a decline in overall mood and motivation, and the onset of injury or infection. Any one of these is all the excuse you need to cancel an interval workout or take a couple of guilt-free days off completely.

Peak Period

If you regard your training program as a pyramid (which is actually a pretty darn good analogy), you're now only a few steps below the very top. You foundation and supporting walls have been built; now it's time to add the needle-sharp point at the very peak.

"Peaking" refers to a state of 100 percent readiness. When you're peaking, you'll ride faster than you ever thought possible, and often it will hardly feel like you're trying. Peaking is when everything comes together. It's a feeling unlike any other, and no small part of why cyclists struggle through dozens of "off" days.

You're now only a few weeks out from your first priority event. The training you're going to complete during the next few weeks is going to be harder than anything you've ever done on a bicycle. Fortunately, it's not going to last long. The efforts you'll use to initiate a peak will be extreme but short, and even as you introduce these efforts, your total training volume will decline.

This 2- to 4-week period is built on power intervals, which are defined as 15- to 30-second efforts that, as Friel delicately puts it, "make

SAMPLE BUILD WEEK »»»

Monday: OFF or short, easy ride below 80% ATHR

Total Duration: 60 minutes

Intensity: Low

Tuesday: Base ride

Total Duration: 60–120 minutes

Intensity: Low-medium (below 88% ATHR)

Wednesday: AE workout as described on previous pages

Total Duration: 60–90 minutes

Intensity: High

Thursday: Base ride

Total Duration: 60–120 minutes

Intensity: Low-medium

Friday: OFF

Saturday: Base ride

Total Duration: 90–180 minutes

Intensity: Low-medium

Sunday: AE workout or base ride

Total Duration: 60–90 minutes

Intensity: High

Total Hours: 6.5–11

you feel like you're going to puke." Thankfully, you'll get maximum recovery after each effort—at least five times the interval length, though more is fine.

And the payoff is commensurate with the pain: These are the intervals that develop the power you'll need to hang with sudden attacks and even initiate a few of your own!

Start with shorter efforts of about 15 seconds, for a total of 6 minutes of interval time over the course of the workout. Do the math and you'll come up with 24 intervals, which might seem like a typographical error, until you consider just how short these efforts are. Add a few seconds to each interval at each subsequent workout, until you're doing 10 minutes total. At the same time, slowly drop your total volume of training. The best way is to decrease the duration of your easy rides (because you're adding interval time to your hard days, you won't be able to cut these shorter). Don't worry about an erosion of fitness. In fact, expect just the opposite: Your body and mind will relish the extra rest and respond by performing at levels greater than ever before.

Again, take a less-is-more approach to this type of interval work. Think of power intervals as tequila: fun in moderation but a heck of a lot of trouble if you overdo it. You cannot be too careful with this sort of high-intensity work. If you've followed the program and don't have any extenuating life circumstances, you should flourish with carefully metered power interval workouts. But if anything's out of whack, you'll be prone to the ravages of overtraining. At this point, with your priority event only a few weeks (or less) away, you can't afford that.

Recovery Weeks

If we listed these workouts in order of importance, this section would come first. That's because without proper recovery, you're going to go nowhere. And fast.

Still, a recovery week is not a week off. Instead, it's a riding week carefully calibrated to allow your body and mind to dump fatigue and rebuild for the training to come. You'll still do one hard workout in the middle of the week, but you should perform only about half as many efforts as usual. The remainder of your week should consist of low- to medium-intensity rides at approximately 60 percent of your normal duration. This schedule should allow adequate recovery while keeping your systems "alive" and ready for more arduous training. If after a full week of reduced volume and intensity you're not champing at the bit or if your overtraining markers are active, continue with the recovery program until things turn around. It's been said before, but it's worth saying again: Never let your planned training schedule preside over your physical and mental state. Always, always allow yourself the flexibility to take time off if your body and brain are asking for it.

The Smart Schedule

Joe Friel understands the scheduling challenges faced by amateur riders who simply can't carve out large chunks of weekday time for training. That's why he often imposes an alternative to the 7-days-make-a-week training schedule. "Sometimes, I'll design a schedule that's 9 days on and 5 days off," explains Friel. "This allows riders to complete their recovery period during the workweek and take advantage of the weekends before and after for hard training."

Of course, 5 days is fewer than 7, so if you plan to tinker with your training schedule in this manner, it's absolutely critical that you monitor yourself carefully to ensure you're getting enough rest. The point is that there's nothing sacrilegious in tweaking your training schedule to fit your lifestyle. Most training schedules are built around a 7-day week simply for convenience's sake, not because there's anything magical about 7 days. Take a close look at your schedule and habits, and don't be afraid to adjust your training based on what you find.

Getting Specific

Success on this (or any) program demands specificity. That is, you need to tailor your training to your priority events.

The easiest and best way to do this is to train on terrain and equipment that closely approximate those events. For instance, if your first

SAMPLE POWER INTERVAL WEEK >>>>>

Monday: OFF

Tuesday: Base ride

Total Duration: 60 minutes

Intensity: Low-medium (below 88% ATHR)

Wednesday: Power interval workout

Total Duration: 60 minutes

Intensity: Very high

Thursday: Base ride

Total Duration: 60–90 minutes

Intensity: Low-medium

Friday: OFF

Saturday: Base ride

Total Duration: 60–90 minutes

Intensity: Low-medium

Sunday: Power interval workout

Total Duration: 60 minutes

Intensity: Very high

Total Hours: 5–6

priority event is a cross-country mountain bike race over rolling terrain, you should do your interval training on short climbs. If it's an individual time trial over roads so flat they'd make a pancake jealous, swing a leg over your time trial bike and head for the flatlands. A road race? Approximate the course in your training.

Of course, this isn't always feasible, and if that's the case for you, don't fret. These workouts can be performed on road and off (though the frequent terrain changes inherent to mountain biking make it difficult to do highly structured interval work), in the hills, or on the flats. Even if you live in Kansas, you can train for a hilly road race by doing your efforts into headwinds or on highway overpasses, or even in parking garages. Be creative and make it fun.

5

SPECIAL GROUP: MOUNTAIN BIKERS

As the sport of mountain biking has evolved, it's become more and more common to find elite-level racers training on the road. Why? "Mountain biking takes a big toll on your body," says Todd Wells, the top U.S. finisher at the 2004 Olympic mountain bike event. "You can do a 1-hour mountain bike ride and get really beat up, or you can go out on the road for an hour and feel like you didn't do anything."

Wells isn't referring to the relative merits of the disciplines as they relate to cardiovascular conditioning; rather, he's talking about the punishment dished out by the rugged terrain that's part and parcel of mountain biking. "When your upper-body muscles are trying to recover from a rugged mountain bike ride, it slows the entire recovery process," says Wells. "You simply can't train as hard."

Still, it's not as if you can simply forgo off-road riding until race day. If you did so, your technical skills would wither, and you'd be off the pace come race day, no matter how fit you were. That's why Wells still does as much as 50 percent of his weekly training on his mountain bike. But, he cautions, "the trails around my home in Durango, Colorado, are really smooth. I can ride them without getting really beat up."

Wells admits that even if training on his mountain bike were detrimental to his performance, he'd probably do it anyway. "I love riding my mountain bike; that's why I got into the sport in the first place. I can't just let go of that. Sometimes, it's more important for me to go out and do the ride that I want to do, rather than the one that might be a little better from a training standpoint."

Wells has another message for eager mountain bikers: Take time off. During the season, when he's racing every weekend (and, sometimes, twice on a weekend), Wells often opts out of any hard training during the week. "It really depends on how much you race," says Wells. "But even if you're racing once a weekend or close to it, you'd be surprised how much recovery you need. Mountain bike races are like 2-hour time trials. Yeah, they're shorter than most road races, but they take a much bigger toll. I think most mountain bike racers, top guys and amateurs, do way too much hard riding during the week."

Another factor to his success is an annual midseason break, during which the Olympian puts his bike in the garage and leaves it to gather dust for 2 weeks. "I just go out and play golf and drink beer," admits Wells. "And when I come off my break, I'm always faster than I was before."

16

THE HEART-RATE TRAP

In this and other training books, you'll see plenty of references to heart rate. That's because it is simply the most accessible way to determine intensity.

But as we mentioned earlier, there are numerous factors that can influence your heart rate and leave you with a false impression of intensity. There's no way around some of these influences, but by examining them and knowing what they are, you can better understand your body and how it responds to both effort and other factors. In fact, once you become tuned in to your heart rate, you'll be able to use it as an early-warning sign to help you ward off illness or overtraining.

The first step is simple: Wear your monitor every time you ride. Interestingly enough, many seasoned pros don't wear their monitors on every ride, but that's because they've become so keyed in to their body's response to effort that they can effectively train by "feel." You should also allow "feel" (some people call it "perceived exertion") to guide your training, but in the early stages of your competitive cycling career, it's good to have another marker to rely on, and the more you monitor your heart rate, the more you'll begin to see correlations between it and external factors.

What are these factors? Well, caffeine is a common one. We all know the sweaty-palms, flutter-chest feeling that comes with too much coffee (heck, that's why some of us drink it in the first place). That's because caffeine stimulates the central nervous system, leading to an increase in both resting and active heart rates. Caffeine is a heart-rate double whammy because it's also a diuretic; another cause of fluctuating heart rate is dehydration. Does this mean you should give up coffee and other foods (think chocolate) that contain caffeine? Of course not. But like any drug (yes, caffeine is a drug), it can be dangerous and detrimental to your health if used unwisely. So long as you don't exceed a cup or three a day, you should be fine.

Of course, training can actually reduce your heart rate. That's because your heart is a muscle, and like any muscle, it grows and becomes more powerful with use. As your fitness improves, you'll notice a decrease in resting heart rate (your heart rate immediately upon waking in the morning, before getting out of bed) and the heart rate it takes to maintain a given workload. These decreases are very good signs that your training is having the desired effect.

If, on the other hand, your resting heart rate increases (you should get in the habit of checking and recording it each morning), you should suspect a couple of things. One, you might be on the edge of overtraining, and two, you might be on the edge of getting sick. In either case, the remedy is the same: Back off until your resting heart rate returns to normal.

Other factors that can affect heart rate include medications (if you're on any type of medication, check with your doc before diving into an exercise regimen), increases in altitude, hot weather, and life stress.

For all these reasons, relying on heart rate as a training gauge can become a dangerous pitfall. At the same time, once you've become intimately familiar with your heart-rate response to both exercise and various external factors, you can use fluctuations in heart rate to better understand what's happening in your body and life. For instance, most athletes find that when they're fit and well-rested, they can raise their heart rates to high levels quickly and with relative ease. But when hard efforts fail to create the typical heart-rate response, it's often a sign of impending illness or overtraining. Of course, everyone has a slightly different response to these factors, so it's important to track your heart rate and perceived exertion until you fully understand how they relate.

17

RECOVERY

An entire chapter devoted to recovery? This book is supposed to be about training on a bike; what's recovery got to do with it? Well, listen up: "Probably the most important factor in a cyclist's progress is his or her ability to recover properly," says Rick Crawford, a cycling coach based in Durango, Colorado. "And it's probably the most overlooked factor." There you have it.

The basic problem is this: Cycling is a hard sport, and competitive cyclists are hard people accustomed to pain and suffering. In fact, this is why many are attracted to the sport in the first place. That's all well and good, but all the suffering in the world won't make you a better cyclist if you don't allow for proper recovery. Remember: When you train, you're actually destroying muscle tissue. It's during the recovery period that it regenerates, coming back stronger than before.

To the committed cyclist, recovery should factor into everything they do off the bike. It should dictate how and when they eat, sleep, and relax. There's an old cycling saying that goes like this: Never run when you can walk, never walk when you can stand, never stand when you can sit, and never sit when you can lie down. This helps explain why professional cyclists do little else besides train, eat, and sleep. Daily naps and massages are the rule, rather than the exception, and during the peak of training and racing, household duties are left to supportive spouses or hired help. Sounds nice, huh? But for most of us, such a cycle-centric lifestyle is about as realistic as a weekend jaunt to Mars. Still, there's plenty you can do to improve recovery, even within the boundaries of a busy off-the-bike life.

First, consider what you can do on the bike to effect recovery. The most important thing is consuming adequate carbohydrates so you don't dig yourself too deep a hole. This means filling your water bottles with sports drink for any rides longer than 60 minutes and stocking your jersey pockets with snacks and energy gels. Shoot for about 300 calories per hour, from a source that has a carbohydrate-to-protein ratio of approximately 4:1, the ideal ratio for keeping glycogen stocked and muscles fed. After long rides (over 90 minutes), make sure to replenish your glycogen stores within 30 minutes with a high-carb snack (or meal, if it's mealtime).

Another on-the-bike recovery trick is making sure to include a proper cooldown at the end of your ride. This should be comprised of 20 minutes of easy spinning at a high (100 to 110 rpm) cadence, which helps flush lactic acid from your muscles. If possible, after particularly hard training days or races, it's valuable to spend 15 to 30 minutes spinning in the evening. This is best done on an indoor trainer, both because it's more time efficient and because it's easier to monitor your effort.

Naps: Whenever you can steal a nap, do so, even if it's only 20 minutes. Sleep is crucial to the production of growth hormone, which is a huge factor in increasing strength and fitness (that's why some athletes resort to illegal doping with growth hormone).

Massage: Can't afford regular massages? Then perform self-massage by elevating your legs and working downward, making sure to hit the calves, hamstrings, and quads. Even a few minutes a day can make a big difference. And if you can afford it, by all means get a professional massage, even if it's only a few times over the course of the season. Try to schedule them so they fall the day after a hard training session or race.

Stay hydrated: Keep a water bottle at your desk and in your car, and sip from it frequently. Monitor your urine; if it's not clear or pale yellow, drink more.

Avoid alcohol: A glass of wine with dinner isn't going to hurt anything (and may even help; red wine is rich in antioxidants), but drinking to the point of inebriation will. Save your imbibing for the off-season.

Eat right: But you knew that, right?

Deal with stress: Don't let nagging life stresses accumulate and grow. When stress pops up (as it invariably will), use your problem-solving skills to counter it and move on. Harboring stressful situations and dwelling on stress is a recovery killer and will have a hugely negative impact on your training.

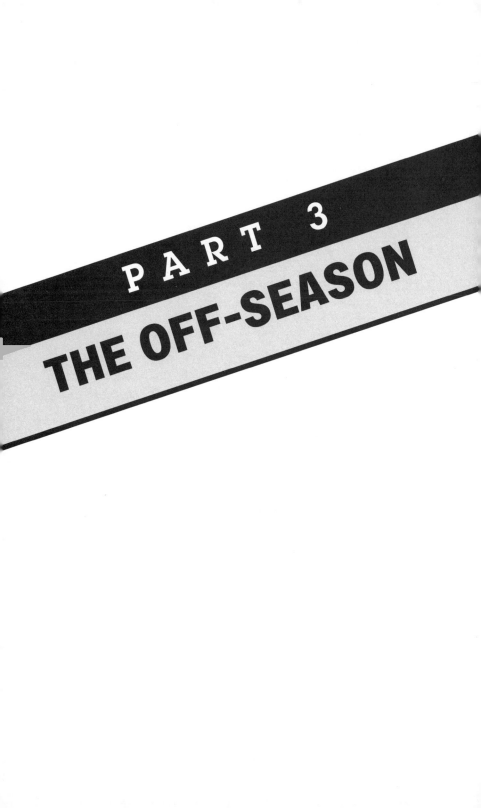

PART 3
THE OFF-SEASON

A journalist once asked Lance Armstrong when he began preparations for the Tour de France. His reply? The day after the previous Tour ends. That's an exaggeration, of course (even Lance celebrates), but it illustrates an important training truth: The "off-season" is a crucial part of your training program.

Granted, you're not gunning for the top spot in the Tour de France (well, okay, maybe you are), but even so, you can take a lesson from the champ's approach. The key is to properly balance your physical and mental regeneration from the previous season with the physical and mental preparation necessary for the coming season. It's a tricky mix, and one that even the sport's top riders struggle with.

Much of how you approach the off-season depends on how you feel going into the off-season. This is pretty easy to figure out: Are you still excited about training and racing? Or do you have to poke yourself in the butt with a sharp stick just to get out the door and on your bike? In either scenario, you should plan to take some time away from the bike, but if it's the latter, you need to plan some serious downtime.

Most serious cyclists begin the off-season with a complete break from the bike. This is good even if you're still physically and mentally motivated: Remember, it's only a matter of weeks until you begin serious off-season training, and if you don't take a break now, you might be very sorry later. And missing training time later could have a negative impact on your performances next year.

If you're still firing on all cylinders, you might want to postpone your break to take advantage of your fitness and motivation. Consider entering some cyclocross races. Cyclocross, with its manic blend of riding, running, and hurdling, is a great way to hone your bike-handling skills and hone top-end fitness. The races are short, ranging from 30 to 60 minutes, so you don't need a tremendous amount of endurance to participate. All you need is a 'cross bike (a mountain bike will do in a pinch) and a whole bunch of gumption. Many professional road and mountain bike racers spend October, November, and December tackling the 'cross circuit.

If you're running on fumes, don't worry: You're not alone. And don't stress: Next season is many, many months away. A few weeks off the bike will only do you good. If you feel like being active in other ways, go for it, with one caveat: Don't jump into other activities with reckless abandon, or injury may soon follow. This is particularly true of weight-bearing sports like running, which has caused many an inflamed tendon or ligament among cross training cyclists. This is a good time to go on hikes with the family, play soccer with the kids, and generally goof off. If you feel like doing nothing, that's fine, too. What's important is taking a break from your bike and following your heart.

Assuming you've following a traditional seasonal schedule, this break is probably taking place in late October and early November. Depending on where you live, your return to training may be accompanied by snow or, at the very least, icy winds and rain. For a top professional, who needs to begin base mile training at this point, this would be a problem. But for amateur cyclists—even elite amateurs—winter is a fantastic opportunity to pursue other sports.

18

CROSS-COUNTRY SKIING

Three-time Tour de France winner Greg LeMond was famous for his Nordic-skiing exploits, which included regular 4- and 5-hour outings across the snow-covered wilderness around his Minnesota home. While most of us can't find the time to ski for 5 hours straight (nor do we need to), we all can benefit from cross-country skiing, which utilizes many of the same muscles as cycling and is reputed to be the best fitness-boosting sport in the world.

There are two basic styles of cross-country skiing. You're probably most familiar with the striding "classic," or "diagonal," technique, which usually takes place in set tracks at a cross-country ski center.

But the more modern skate technique has become very popular among cyclists, for a number of reasons.

1. It's easier to learn.

2. It doesn't demand complicated and labor-intensive waxing.

3. It's incredibly physically demanding and can boost fitness in a very short period of time (in fact, you need to be really, really careful to avoid overtraining when skate skiing).

Either classic or skate skiing can comprise the bulk of your off-season cross training. If you live in a snowy climate, consider implementing a cross-country ski program that closely mimics your in-season cycling schedule in frequency, duration, and intensity. You'll still need to spend the first couple months of the cycling season in base mileage mode, but once that's completed, you'll be drawing on a deep well of fitness. And the time spent on skis is time spent off the bike, which will only grow your hunger for turning the pedals.

19

ALPINE SKIING

At first glance, alpine skiing would appear to have little to do with cycling. And while it's true that gliding downhill on a pair of fancy planks won't do much for your cardiovascular fitness, it's also true that lift-serviced skiing has much to recommend it. Not convinced? Consider that Olympic alpine champion Hermann Maier, perhaps the greatest alpine skier in the long history of the sport, is renowned for his strength on the bike.

The key is to ski like Hermann does, which is, in a word, aggressively. When Maier clicks into his bindings, he's not looking for a mellow day on the slopes with his buddies. Instead, he charges run after run, carving hard, fast turns that force him to engage his glutes and quads in way that's similar to cycling. The benefit to his cycling? Greater power.

Alpine skiing is also appealing simply because it's fun, and we can all do with more of that. There's nothing quite like charging down a powder-cloaked slope on a pristine winter's day. However, because it doesn't provide much of a boost to your aerobic fitness, you'll need to supplement heavily with other cross training or with riding itself.

20 >>>

RUNNING

Running is the world's most popular fitness tool for a number of reasons. For one, it's cheap (all you need are a pair of socks and running shoes, although your neighbors would probably appreciate it if you wore shorts or tights also). For another, it doesn't demand a heck of a lot of skill. And finally, like all weight-bearing activities, it's brutally efficient. A 40-minute run can deliver a wallop of fitness.

Still, running carries some significant caveats. Chief among them is injury, and this is particularly true for fit cyclists who strap on a pair of shoes and try to run up to their fitness. In other words, their cardiovascular systems are well-developed, but their running musculature is not, leaving them prone to injury. The other problem with running is that the fitness you glean simply doesn't carry over very well to cycling. This isn't a big deal in the early phases of the off-season, but as winter progress, you'll need to add more cycling-specific exercise to your routine.

This doesn't mean you should give up on running; it merely means you need to be considered in your approach. Start very slowly: 10 minutes is not too short for your first run. Run only every other day, upping your time by 10 percent on each outing. Try to avoid pavement, which is harsh on your knees and ankles. Instead, stick to gravel roads and trails. For an interesting change of perspective, run the trails you usually ride on your mountain bike.

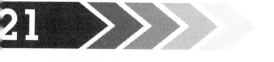

WEIGHT TRAINING

Until the 1980s, cyclists rarely lifted weights. In fact, weight training was spurned by most endurance athletes, and the physique of choice was the marathoning ideal—lean to the point of emaciation. Few cyclists had weight training experience, and most coaches didn't believe it could help riders improve. Iron was anathema.

But now, in one of training theory's periodic about-faces, everyone is pumping iron enthusiastically. What happened? On the recreational side, cyclists got tired of wimpy-looking upper bodies. Buffness became cool. (It's probably no coincidence that the move to weight training coincided with the popularity of form-fitting spandex.) Vanity aside, the Eastern European cyclists of the 1980s demonstrated that with strength came speed. The great East German and Soviet sprinters were built like Greek gods.

For long-distance riders, weight training became a way to condition the upper body for the rigors of hours in the saddle. It was thought that the best way to do this was simply to ride, and the arms, shoulders, neck, and back would adapt. Cyclists now realize that weights can effectively build the required strength, making the season's first long rides more comfortable and allowing endurance to improve at a faster rate.

Despite this new enthusiasm for weight training, however, findings from the National Strength and Conditioning Association indicate that some cyclists are going about it in ways that may be less effective than they could be. Circuit training, high repetitions, endless squats—all have their outspoken advocates.

But there are other valid methods. What should you do? Read about them and use the information to design a workout routine that suits your enthusiasm and time for weight training as well as your cycling objectives. Much more important than which approach you follow is that you make weight training part of your program.

Strength and Aerobic Power

Most people used to think that cyclists were aerobic athletes, shot-putters were strength athletes, and never the twain should meet. But now the word is out that max VO_2—the lab test that measures maximal oxygen consumption and indicates cycling potential—is inseparable from leg strength. For proof, recall a day when your legs were tired from several consecutive hard rides, and no matter how hard you tried, you couldn't elevate your heart rate. If you had taken a max VO_2 test, the results would have been far below your potential.

Now suppose your legs felt fresh but lacked strength. You'd experience the same disheartening results. "If your legs are too weak to drive your heart and lungs to maximum levels, your max VO_2 performance will be low," explains David Martin, exercise physiology researcher at the Olympic Training Center in Colorado Springs. "Strengthen the legs and you can improve your peak VO_2 and your cycling performance."

Peter Francis, Ph.D., renowned for his work in cycling biomechanics, agrees with this basic change in training philosophy. "The traditional approach to cycling was to ride a great deal," he says. "Now we believe that cycling inefficiently only trains you to cycle inefficiently. We know that specific strength training is important."

Injury Prevention

The benefit of strength training is vital to racers and recreational riders who don't want the loss of fitness and health that injuries cause. Weight training strengthens the shoulder girdle and neck, helping you withstand overuse injuries and absorb crash impacts. A good leg program balances the strength of the opposing muscles (quadriceps and hamstrings) to help you avoid muscle pulls from hard efforts. Weight training is your injury insurance policy. You need to lift wisely, however, or weight training won't insure against injury; it will ensure that you suffer one. Moderation is key to improvement and avoiding an injury in the weight room. Cyclists who don't overdo "iron therapy" don't lose their freshness, either.

"The difference between fitness and fatigue is performance," says Martin. If your legs are dead from too much strength work, you won't benefit from time on the bike. Furthermore, he says, there's no need to fear loss of conditioning as you rest, since "fatigue is eliminated faster than fitness."

Remember, there's no cycling-related reason to build bulging biceps, and a 400-pound deadlift is useful only in hoisting your bike onto the roof rack (and only if your bike weighs a heck of a lot more than it should). "Don't waste time doing more than necessary in the weight room," stresses Harvey Newton, a masters racer and a former U.S. Olympic weight lifting coach. "Get in, do a cycling-specific strength workout, and then go on to something else."

The late Carl Leusenkamp, a national-team track coach, used to remind his riders, "Don't let weight training become an end in itself. Use weights to help you go faster on the bike." If you're a committed cyclist, those words of wisdom should be with you every minute you're in the weight room.

Proper Planning

Early attempts at incorporating weight training into cycling programs often failed because they were badly planned. Know what you want from strength training before you begin. Each fall, formulate your goals for the coming year. "Look at the end of the riding season as the beginning of your year," advised Leusenkamp. "Evaluate and plan." A valuable tool is a training diary, which helps you assess your performance and stay motivated.

Athletes in all sports vary their training to avoid staleness and create periods of performance. "You need a long-range, year-round approach to training," explains Newton, "because a cyclist has only about 4 months to do serious strength training." He suggests starting in October with a transitional weight training phase lasting about 4 weeks. By varying the exercises, by using light weights with a greater number of repetitions, and by working out two or three times per week, you'll accustom your muscles to lifting.

Ease gradually from riding to weight training because, as Dr. Francis warns, "the best predictor of injury is change."

Next comes a 4- to 6-week "hypertrophy," or preliminary strength building, period. It features thrice-weekly workouts using three sets of each exercise done for 8 to 12 repetitions apiece. Both of these early phases are vital. "If you begin strength training without transitional and hypertrophy periods," warns Newton, "you'll get injured."

Only then are you ready for the meat of the program: 4 to 6 weeks of basic strength development, using five or more sets of each exercise, with no more than eight reps apiece. Conclude with a month of power development by doing three or four sets of exercises specific to cycling (leg presses, stepups, lunges) and using slightly higher reps (about 15) and greater speed of movement.

Afterward, don't let your hard-earned strength deteriorate during the riding season. Maintain it with pushups, pullups, and abdominal exercises at least twice a week. But don't forget that your priority is cycling. "When the season begins, it's not the time to set records in the weight room," says Newton.

Reconsidering Traditional Ways

When planning your training, don't repeat the mistakes of the past. For example, calf raises have traditionally been part of cycling weight programs. After all, when you ride behind someone with impressive calves, it looks as if they're vital to the pedal stroke. But "it's the quads that are actually flexing the foot," says Dr. Francis. "The calf muscles act merely as a tight wire to transfer the quads' power to the foot and pedal." So, forgo the calf raises and focus on developing the quad power that really counts.

Circuit training has been similarly misinterpreted. It involves a series of light-weight/high-repetition exercises aimed at building muscle endurance and cardiovascular fitness. Recent research, however, indicates that its effect on aerobic fitness is minimal, especially for athletes who already are conditioned by endurance sports such as cycling. Because of this, Newton recommends using weights for their primary purpose: improving strength. "I recommend three to five sets of about 10 reps rather than high-rep training or circuits," he says.

There's no reason to spend hours in the weight room, even in midwinter. Six exercises packed into 30 minutes are all you need. Do an exercise for the quads, such as leg presses or stepups, and leg curls for the hamstrings. Choose an upper-body pulling movement, such as bent-over rows, and a pushing exercise, such as bench presses. Then add two "assistance" exercises, such as abdominal crunches and back extensions. "Cyclists use lower-back muscles to keep from straightening up on powerful pedal strokes," explains Dr. Francis. "They also need strong abdominals to avoid back injuries."

One-Set Theory

Here's good news if you're a recreational cyclist simply looking for better muscle balance and tone, along with some injury protection. Because you're not seeking maximum development from weight training, you can do just one set of each exercise and still get good results while saving time and energy.

Sure, it sounds like an empty promise, but that's the recent finding of researchers Ralph Carpinetti and Robert Otto, who say that in 33 of 35 studies, there was "no significant difference in strength increase between individuals performing single-set and those performing multiple-set exercise." Their conclusion: Doing 1 set of four to six exercises, each with 8 to 12 reps, provides nearly the same benefit as doing 2 or more (up to as many as 15) sets of each exercise. If this method sounds good to you, use a weight that allows all reps in good form. When you can exceed 12 reps, increase the weight by about 3 percent.

Naturally, there are dissenters. Newton, for instance, points out that while single-set routines did work well in studies that lasted 8 to 12 weeks, multiple sets are more effective over the longer duration of a typical winter program. There's also the warmup factor. Doing at least two sets lets you use a lighter weight the first time through before using the optimal weight.

Researcher Everett Harmon, Ph.D., advocates three sets total, contending that "muscles seem to need preparation to go all-out. Doing two preliminary sets of about 80 and 90 percent of the final weight works better."

The bottom line? If your energy, workout time, or interest in weight training is limited and your choice is between a minimal program and no program at all, go the one-set route. There will be noticeable improvement for the few minutes you spend each week. On the other hand, if you have the time and ambition, you should see even greater benefits from a multiple-set program.

Tips from a Top Coach

The Bulgarians have long been at the forefront of strength development. Their lifters have won Olympic and world titles disproportionate to their country's population, and their coaches have become leaders in applying the principles of strength development to other sports. Bulgarian national weight lifting coach Angel Spassov often offers advice for cyclists during lecture tours.

Be Patient

Weight training is not a quick fix. Three weeks or even 3 months in the weight room won't elevate you from a century rider to Paris–Brest–Paris champion. "You need 6 to 8 years of training to be world class in any sport," says Spassov. Your body will improve, but only on its own timetable. Forcing rapid improvement in cycling or weight training leads to injury, stalled progress, and staleness. "Always, when we break the laws of nature," he says, "we make mistakes."

Use Technology

The same heart-rate monitor that's so valuable for training on the bike is also useful for winter weight workouts. When riding, you elevate your heart rate to near maximum during interval training and let it drop to about 120 beats per minute for recovery. Nearly the same principles apply to strength training. "In power sports," explains Spassov, "strength is best built in the 160-to-180 range. But let your heart rate drop much lower between sets."

Use Weights to Develop Cycling-Specific Strength

Doing intervals up steep hills builds power. But so do leg presses—and they do it faster. "It's hard to use your sport to develop power to its fullest," says Spassov. "If you use an aerobic sport, it takes much longer. You need weights." For endurance cyclists, this supports the contention that upper-body strength can be developed better in the weight room than on the bike. Bench presses, rows, crunches, and back extensions are particularly effective at conditioning the muscles likely to fatigue during long rides.

Be Aware of the Link

Endurance doesn't exist separately from strength. For example, Spassov explains that a runner takes about 27,000 steps during a marathon and, with each step, pushes two times his body weight. That's about 1,600 tons over the 26 miles, so the need for strength is evident. In addition, Spassov maintains that while the marathon runner's heart rate returns to normal about 3 hours after the event and the blood profile is back at baseline in 3 days, the legs need about a month to recover. The more strength the legs possess, the faster the recovery.

Keep Resistance Low to Maintain Speed and Technique

Work with 28 percent of your one-rep maximum to build endurance, Spassov recommends. For instance, if you can bench-press

150 pounds one time, do multiple reps with 40 pounds to build endurance.

Step Up to Stepups

Squats have long been the cornerstone of strength programs, but they are no longer done in the Bulgarian system. "Squats put too much compression on the lower back," explains Spassov, "and there's no correlation between squat performance and sports performance." As a result, he substitutes a related exercise called stepups. This alternative is effective for the legs but easier on the back. Here's how to do it.

1. Face a bench. It should be high enough so that your thigh is parallel to the ground when you put a foot on it and stand on the toes of your rear foot.

2. Step up onto the bench. Don't push off with your rear leg; make sure the leg on the bench does all the work. Staying on the toes of your rear leg will ensure that it doesn't get involved.

3. Don't alternate legs after each rep. Instead, keep the same leg on the bench until you have done the planned number of reps; then switch legs.

4. Start the exercise using just your body weight as resistance. As you get stronger, hold a barbell or an inner tube filled with sand over your shoulders. Don't use more weight than your maximum squat or leg-press weight divided by 2.2.

Mix Weight Training and Cycling

In the early season, do easy warmups of 15 minutes on the bike or resistance trainer, followed by several intervals of hard pedaling mixed with easy pedaling, Spassov recommends. Then get off the bike, change shoes, and do a short, intense program of leg development, including stepups and leg presses. Get back on the bike and spin easily for 15 minutes to cool down. Mixing cycling and weight training in the same workout ensures that the strength you're building transfers to the specific movement of cycling. You'll keep your pedaling finesse as you get stronger.

2.2

INDOOR RIDING

It's been said so often, it's almost a cycling cliché: The best training for riding is . . . riding. That's why professional cyclists spend 3 or 4 weeks at most off the bike each year. There is simply no substitute for turning the pedals. That's great news if you live in, say, Florida. But if you're reading this in front of a crackling wood fire at your mountain retreat in Montana, it's not exactly what you want to hear.

Now, remember, you're not a pro. For even elite-level amateurs, long periods of cross training are not only adequate; they may be preferable simply because time off the bike is refreshing to both body and mind. But even cross training converts can benefit from regular rides on an indoor trainer or rollers. This is especially true as the off-season wanes. Depending on your goals for the season, you may need to begin base miles when winter's fury is at its peak. And while riding through the snow and sleet is possible (and occasionally even fun), at some point you're going to have to look inward.

Indoor riding holds other advantages, too. You're not dependent on daylight, for one. And riding in a controlled environment (such as your basement) makes it that much easier to gauge your efforts and ensure you're getting just what you need from the workout.

The key to successful indoor riding is contained in two words: diversion and variety. To satisfy the former, create a riding environment rich in entertainment. The ideal setup would include a big-screen TV, a half dozen or so speakers, and a DVD player. That may not be feasible, but if you're planning to rack up some serious indoor miles, a DVD player or VCR is worth its weight in gold. Headphones will ensure you don't wake up the family or neighbors. Music is a good friend, too, and some riders rig book or magazine supports on their handlebars.

One key component to successful indoor riding that's often neglected is a fan. Even if you set up in a cool spot like your basement, you're going to create a heck of a lot of heat. Set up a fan that you can reach from your bike so you can adjust its speed as your ride progresses. If you stay cool and comfy, you'll ride more efficiently and be more likely to grunt through the final miles of a ride you might otherwise end early.

Trainer or Rollers?

Perhaps the biggest question indoor riding newbies face is whether to pursue their passion on a stationary trainer or rollers, which are free-rolling drums that closely mimic the feel of outdoor riding.

To decide, consider what you want to accomplish. Because stationary trainers require no particular skill to ride and because you'd have to try very hard to tip over while clamped into one, they're the best pick for inexperienced riders or anyone who just wants to get on and zone out. It's also much easier to do sprint workouts on a trainer simply because there's no risk of crashing.

Rollers, on the other hand, will help you develop a silky spin and improve your bike-handling skills. That's because on rollers you're on your own. Just like in the real world, you can fall while riding rollers. In fact, every serious roller rider has a roller tale of woe that typically involves—pick one—a coffee table, a hardwood floor, or a china cabinet. But rollers have another, lesser-known advantage. Because they demand a certain level of mental engagement, time seems to pass more quickly. And for what it's worth, roller proficiency is a cycling rite of passage. When you can ride your rollers no-handed, you're a serious cyclist, no matter what your results say.

Keep It Short

No matter what you ride, or what you watch or listen to while riding, keep your indoor rides short. The idea is to keep your legs accustomed to the bike, not put the finishing touches on your peaking program. It's not that indoor training can't accomplish this, but remember: It's the off-season. Save it for warmer days. Instead, let your cross training take care of your overall fitness, and use indoor cycling as a way to stay in touch with the bike. Three or four short (30- to 50-minute) rides per week are plenty, and even two will make a big difference when the weather warms. With a few indoor miles in your legs, your cycling-specific fitness will come around much more

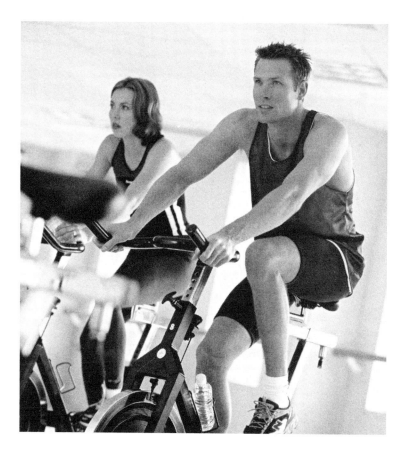

quickly, and you'll be much less likely to suffer an overuse injury when you start racking up the miles.

Instead, use indoor training to work on improving your spin and increasing pedaling efficiency. One of the best ways to do this is with one-legged pedaling drills (this is much easier on a stationary trainer, though experience roller riders are encouraged to give it a shot). Once you've warmed up thoroughly, clip one foot out of its pedal and keep spinning with the other leg. You'll need to use a very small gear, and you'll be amazed at how quickly you fatigue, a symptom of inefficiency that should improve with these workouts. Start with as few as 25 revolutions before switching sides. Do five sets of these; then cool down. On each subsequent indoor ride, add 5 revolutions to each set. Stick with this workout, and you'll be amazed at the silky-smooth pedaling style that will emerge.

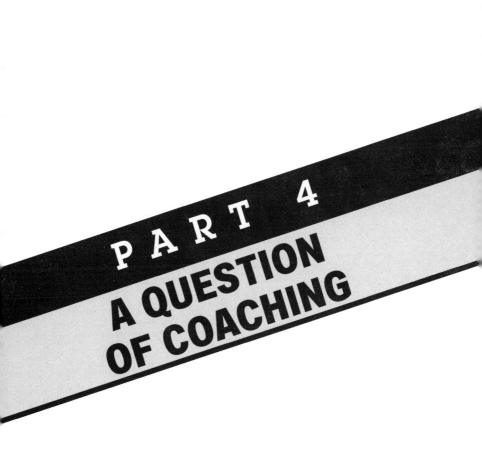

PART 4
A QUESTION OF COACHING

23

THE COACHING CONUNDRUM

Despite the teamwork inherent to road racing, training for cycling remains largely an individual pursuit. Perhaps that helps explain why cyclists tend to be self-taught and self-coached. Most riders rely on training lore and books such as this one to craft a program.

For many, that's not a bad thing. But increasingly cyclists are turning to coaches to guide them through the complexities of designing and implementing a training program. It's a trend spurred in no small part by Lance Armstrong's public relationship with his coach, Chris Carmichael, whose business, Carmichael Training Systems, has evolved to include the coaching of professional sports teams and corporations.

So, should you consider hiring a coach? According to Joe Friel, a top cycling coach and author of *Cyclist's Training Bible*, who counts numerous national champions among his clients, that depends largely on your circumstances and goals. "The biggest reason athletes come to me is because they don't have enough time," says Friel. "They want me to design a program that will maximize their training hours. If someone only has 6 hours a week to train, they can't afford to make mistakes with their program. It needs to be spot-on if they're going to be competitive."

Friel suggests conducting an honest evaluation of your riding and how you view your training. "The athletes that benefit most from coaching are the ones that can't look at themselves objectively," says Friel. "And most athletes can't." For this very reason, it may be helpful to enlist a training partner to help assess your situation.

A coach's most important task is to act as an objective overseer of your training. A good coach will spot the symptoms of overtraining long before you even think to consider it and will adjust your training accordingly. A good coach will keep you motivated and fresh, both by offering outside motivation and by keeping your program from growing stale. A good coach is a shoulder to cry on when things go wrong and someone to celebrate with when they go right.

"It's been a world of difference," says Ralph Heath, who enlisted Friel in January 2004. At 53, Heath had been competing in road races and triathlons for nearly 20 years and had "read probably every training book on the market and every magazine article that was ever published." But all the printed words in the world couldn't do what Friel could. "I understood the concept of periodization," says Heath, the president of a marketing firm. "But planning it out always made me want to take a nap."

Under Friel's guidance, Heath began a highly structured program that saw him training approximately the same number of hours, but at an overall lower intensity. "After 6 or 8 weeks, I noticed I was creeping toward the front during group rides," says Heath. "I was hanging with the big dogs on the climbs. It made me realize that I'd always been overtrained."

In fact, Heath credits his new approach to winning a long-standing battle with exercise-induced asthma. "I think my body was always so run-down that it couldn't keep the asthma at bay. Now it's a nonissue."

The downside? Primarily cost. Although you can probably find someone to coach you for free or next to free, Friel cautions that it's a classic case of "you get what you pay for." For instance, if you want to hire Friel, be prepared to part with $1,000 per month. But Friel also works with numerous "associate" coaches that follow his principles and benefit from his research, while Carmichael Training Systems offers numerous coaching "packages" that start at less than $50 per month. The upshot? Do some research, and you'll find a coach that's a perfect match for your personality, goals, and budget.

24

COACHES' TEST

Okay, so how do you know if you've found the right coach? Like most human connections, it's more art than science, but it's also important to ask a few questions.

With this book under your belt, you should be able to ask the informed questions that will help determine your potential coach's level of expertise. Still, be sure to ask for at least two referrals, and listen very carefully to what they have to say. Also, it's important to be very clear on how often you'll have personal contact with your coach and whether it will be via telephone or e-mail. E-mail is fine for regular updates, but nothing beats telephone (or, if you're lucky enough to live within driving distance, face-to-face) meetings. That's because once your coach gets to know you, he or she will be able to pick up clues simply by listening to the tone of your voice and subtleties in your words. And actual conversations are much more likely to diverge into subjects that may seem irrelevant but are actually gold mines of insight to an experienced coach.

Ultimately, though, it may boil down to "feel." "The right coach will help you step back and look at your life, on and off the bike," says rising road star Tom Danielson. "They should be almost like a psychiatrist. Training is not just the engine; it's also the head, and there's no way to disconnect them."

25

BEST TIPS FROM TOP COACHES

Still not sure you're ready to commit? We tapped some of the world's top cycling coaches to bring you the best coaching tips money can buy. Of course, these can't and shouldn't replace real, live coaching, but they can be valuable assets to your training.

Massimo Testa, M.D.

Dr. Testa is a pro cycling team physician who has planned training for riders, including the indomitable Lance Armstrong. He is internationally respected for defining the optimal combination of work and rest that pro riders need to maintain form through their grueling 9-month racing season.

1. Get plenty of rest year-round. "I used to prescribe lots of intensity, but maybe the riders were overtrained," says Dr. Testa. "Now I schedule more rest days, along with several easy weeks, during the season. We watch carefully for signs of overtraining, including decreased power and speed; increased recovery time; tactical mistakes, including dumb crashes; digestive trouble; weight loss; anxiety; depression; and a bad attitude. If these signs appear, we modify training.

"Recreational riders can do the same. If you crash or get sick or have bad psychology, you have to take some time off."

2. Work on strength and flexibility, too. "We try to prevent problems by doing abdominal exercises and stretching," Dr. Testa says. "A study has shown that cyclists increase their power by 5 percent merely by stretching the hamstrings because added flexibility means better utilization of the quadriceps. We also change their position on the bike if it's needed. But we never adjust their position during the race season, even if it's bad, because they wouldn't have time to adjust and might get injured.

"In the off-season, we use rollers three to five times a week to improve balance and spin. And we do weight training to restore muscle mass lost during the season. Studies show that Tour de France riders gain body fat during the race because they lose muscle volume, especially in the upper body. Winter is the time to counter that effect. We do three sets of 25 reps at 50 percent of the maximum they can lift in that exercise, followed by two sets of 50 reps at 25 percent of max weight. We use high reps and low weights because when you pedal, you use a small percentage of maximum strength on each stroke. We also ride some climbs of 4 to 6 minutes, pedaling at 50 to 60 rpm to build strength and muscle mass."

Tudor Bompa, Ph.D.

Often called the father of periodization training, Dr. Bompa is a legendary figure among endurance coaches. His theories were the basis for East German and Soviet success in the 1980s, and he advocated weight training for endurance athletes before it became widely accepted. He is a professor at York University in Toronto.

1. Plan to meet your goals, but don't be rigid. "Training regimens must be flexible," says Dr. Bompa. "You have to plan for the total stress load in your life, not just the stress from training. Total stress includes job, family, school. You can't divorce training from other aspects of your life."

2. Watch out for too much intensity. "You only improve if you overload your system with occasional hard training. But overloading often leads to overtraining. If you regenerate with easy rides and rest, you'll supercompensate and be better. Don't think 'hard work.' Instead, think 'intelligent work.' Most North Americans are overtrained. When you're ready, you'll feel good physically and mentally. That's when you should do the big event."

3. Repeat workouts to get a training effect. "If you want to develop endurance for a century ride, start doing a long weekend ride at least 1 month before the event."

4. After a hard session, set aside 30 minutes to regenerate. "Sip a carb replacement drink; lie down with your legs elevated. Relax mentally; maybe take a 15-minute nap. Even if you have to borrow the time from training, you'll recover much faster."

5. Heavy weights deserve another look. "I've seen some preliminary results on a track pursuiter who weighed 154 pounds and shifted to power lifting for 2 years. Then he could squat with more than 500 pounds. When he returned to the bike, his pursuit time decreased by 5 seconds. Although we cannot draw universal conclusions, this example is fascinating."

Chris Carmichael

Carmichael rode professionally with the pioneering 7-Eleven team that launched U.S. cycling into the big time. Later, his vision and drive turned the Olympic Training Center (OTC) into a worldwide leader in training techniques. Still Lance Armstrong's personal coach, and the man Armstrong credits with much of his Tour de France success, Carmichael combines the ability to set broad seasonal goals with minutely planned daily training.

Create a vision statement and set goals. "This is important whether you're an elite rider or preparing to ride your first century," says Carmichael. "A vision statement shouldn't be a bunch of touchy-feely stuff. It's designed to provide a long-term goal and direct your actions and emotions. Before you write it, ask yourself, 'If I were to drop dead tomorrow, what would I want people to say about me?' Then write it down. That's your vision statement.

"For instance, here's the U.S. pro riders' group vision statement: 'One hundred percent prepared physically and mentally to race to the full potential of the entire team.' Then they formulated four goals that would help them achieve that. One, a united and committed team. Two, an organized training plan. Three, a clear and defined race strategy. Four, maintain control and commitment to the vision during unplanned disruptions.

"With these as guidelines, you should be able to set up your own vision and goals. For instance, number four is a great goal for every recreational rider who has to deal with a job and family."

Dean Golich

Golich, a cycling coach in Colorado Springs, made his mark with hard work and careful attention to detail. As the recorder and analyzer of the day-to-day training and exercise intensities of national-team riders, he accumulated a wealth of on-bike information. His secret weapon? He's a strong cyclist himself and was able to keep up with the team on most of their training rides to monitor their performances.

1. Ride the machine. "The following ergometer test, devised by the OTC sports-science and -technology division, is a quick way to track your fitness from one month to the next or compare your power to other riders," says Golich. "We often use it to screen riders. You need an ergometer that measures power output in watts. Check at a health club or university human-performance lab. The CompuTrainer, which we use at the OTC, has this feature. If you aren't interested in comparing yourself to others, you can use a resistance trainer and simply increase your gears instead of the watts. After a good warmup, do the following progression."

0 to 3 minutes at 110 watts

3 to 6 minutes at 180 watts

6 to 9 minutes at 250 watts

9 to 12 minutes at 340 watts

12 to 15 minutes at 410 watts

15 to 18 minutes at 480 watts

"These figures are for a 6-foot, 155-pound rider. If you are larger or smaller, increase or decrease watts proportionally. Keep your cadence at 90 rpm. When it falls below 90 for more than 10 seconds, the test is over. This is an all-out test, so check with your doctor before attempting it.

"Elite national-class male riders usually score over 15 minutes for seniors and over 13 for juniors. Women are generally 15 to 20 percent lower. In a similar test, former Olympic champion and pro racer Olaf Ludwig pounded out 600 watts."

2. Make full use of race data. "If you have a heart-rate monitor that stores information for downloading, wear it during a race or competitive ride. Then compare your maximum heart rate and other information with the data collected during training. Most of our riders find that in competition they can reach a higher heart rate and time trial for extended periods at a higher heart rate than they can in training. When we know that, we can reset their training zones."

3. Know your body. "People say that an elevated morning heart rate means you're overtrained. This is a good indicator for some riders. But I've seen other riders have their best races when their heart rates were 10 percent higher than normal."

Hennie Top

A leading Dutch racer in the early 1980s, Top served as U.S. national women's road coach in the 1990s. She is respected as a master of tactics and strategy.

1. Climb at your own pace. "Don't let others dictate your effort. If you aren't a good climber, try to start a long climb at the front of the group and slide gradually to the back as the climb progresses. Maybe you can hang on over the top. Even when you are riding alone, don't go so hard that you blow up halfway up the hill. You won't be able to recover on the descent."

2. If you lose time on climbs, make it up on descents. "Follow an experienced rider down the hill, but don't follow too closely, in case she makes a mistake and crashes. Also, keep your legs going around so they don't stiffen up for the next climb."

Jeff Broker, Ph.D.

Broker, an assistant professor in biomechanics at the University of Colorado in Colorado Springs, is an expert on pedaling mechanics.

He pioneered the use of the SRM PowerMeter in the United States. This German device allows a cyclist's power output to be measured on the bike in actual riding conditions and is instrumental in calculating aerodynamic drag forces for time trialists.

Better aerodynamics save more time than better pedaling. "It's a myth that riders pull up at the bottom of the pedal stroke sufficiently to unload the pedal," Dr. Broker states. "There's also no scientific evidence that improved pedaling mechanics can shave seconds off your time. In fact, lower-level cyclists often have better form than elite riders. And our studies show that mountain bikers seem to pull through at the bottom of the pedal stroke better than track or road riders. Maybe it's because mountain bikers need uniform power delivery through the whole pedal stroke so they don't lose traction on loose surfaces. Theoretically, better pedaling techniques should make you a better cyclist, but scientifically it doesn't seem to be that important.

"Aerodynamics will make you faster than perfect pedaling style. Here's a great example. Wind tunnel results show that eliminating 10 grams of drag saves 158 feet in a 25-mile time trial. How much is 10 grams? It's the drag created by projecting about 4 inches of a pencil into the air stream. That baggy jersey or upright riding position is costing you minutes."

Roy Knickman

A product of the "class of '84," which included Olympic road champion Alexi Grewal and future pro stars Ron Kiefel and Davis Phinney, Knickman also raced professionally before taking over as U.S. national-team road coach. His advice served as a refreshingly simple closer to the coaching conference.

Don't calculate potential success based on test scores. "When I was 15, I had a max VO2 (maximal oxygen consumption) of 72 and was viewed as the next great American rider. Each year after that, my VO2 numbers decreased even though my results got better. Right after my bronze-medal performance in the 1984 Olympic-team time trial—the strongest I've ever been—I was tested again. My max VO2 was 64."

26 >>>

ROAD RIDING POSITION

Arms: Beware road rider's rigor mortis. Keep your elbows bent and relaxed, to absorb shock and prevent veering when you hit a bump. Keep your arms in line with your body, not splayed to the side, to make a more compact, aerodynamic package.

Upper body/shoulders: The operative words: Be still. Imagine the calories burned by rocking from side to side with every pedal stroke on a 25-mile ride. Use that energy for pedaling. Also, beware of creeping forward on the saddle and hunching your back when tired. Periodically shift to a higher gear and stand to pedal, to prevent stiffness in your hips and back.

Head and neck: Avoid putting your head down, especially when you're tired. Periodically tilt your head from side to side to stretch and relax neck muscles.

Hands: Change hand position frequently to prevent finger numbness and upper-body stiffness. A white-knuckle hold on the handlebar is unnecessary and will produce energy-sapping muscle tension throughout your arms and shoulders. Grasp the drops for descents or high-speed riding, and the brake lever hoods for relaxed cruising. On long climbs, hold the top of the bar to sit upright, and open your chest for easier breathing. When standing, grasp the hoods lightly and gently rock the bike from side to side in synch with your pedal strokes. Always keep your thumbs and a finger of each hand closed around the hoods or bar to prevent losing hold on an unexpected bump.

Handlebar: Bar width should equal shoulder width. Err on the side of a wider one to open your chest for breathing. Some models are available with a large drop (vertical distance) to help big hands fit into the hooks. Position the flat, bottom portion of the bar horizontally or pointed slightly down toward the rear brake.

Brake levers: Levers can be moved around the curve of the bar to

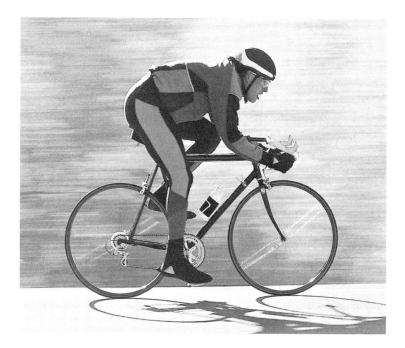

give you the best compromise between holding the hoods and braking when your hands are in the bar hooks. Most riders do best if the lever tips touch a straightedge extended forward from under the flat, bottom portion of the bar.

Stem height: With the stem high enough (normally about an inch below the top of the saddle), you'll be more inclined to use the drops. Putting it lower can improve aerodynamics but may be uncomfortable.

Top tube and stem length: These combined dimensions, which determine your reach, vary according to your flexibility and anatomy. There is no ultimate prescription, but there is a good starting point: When you're comfortably seated with your elbows slightly bent and your hands on the brake hoods, the front hub should be obscured by the handlebar. This is a relatively upright position, and with time you may benefit from a longer stem extension to improve aerodynamics and flatten your back.

Back: A flat back is the defining mark of a pro rider. The correct stem and top tube combination is crucial for this, but so is hip flexibility.

Concentrate on rotating the top of your hips forward. Think of trying to touch the top tube with your stomach. This image will help stop you from rounding your back.

Saddle height: There are various formulas for this, but you needn't be a mathematician to know what the correct height looks like. Your knees should be slightly bent at the bottom of the pedal stroke, and your hips shouldn't rock on the saddle (when viewed from behind). Try this quick method, which is used at the Olympic Training Center in Colorado Springs: Set the height so there is 5 mm of clearance between your heel and the pedal at the bottom of the stroke. Add a few millimeters if your shoes have very thin soles at the heels compared with at the forefeet. Raise the saddle 2 or 3 mm if you have long feet in proportion to your height. For those who have knee pain caused by chondromalacia—a softening or wearing away and cracking of the cartilage under the kneecap that results in pain and inflammation—a saddle on the higher side of the acceptable range can be therapeutic. Gradually raise it until hip rocking begins; then lower it slightly. Make saddle height changes 2 mm at a time to avoid leg strain.

Saddle tilt: The saddle should be level, which you can check by laying a straightedge along its length. A slight downward tilt may be more comfortable if you're using an extreme forward position with an aero bar and elbow rests, but too much causes you to slide forward and place excessive weight on your arms.

Fore/aft saddle position: The trend is to move the saddle back to produce more power for climbing. To start with, sit comfortably in the center of the saddle with the crankarms horizontal. Drop a plumb line from the front of your forward kneecap. It should touch the end of the crankarm. This is the neutral position, and you should be able to achieve it by loosening the seatpost clamp and sliding the saddle fore or aft. Climbers, time trialists, and some road racers prefer the line to fall a couple of centimeters behind the end of the crankarm, to increase leverage in big gears. Conversely, track and criterium racers like a more forward position, to improve leg speed. Remember, if your reach to the handlebar is wrong, use stem length, not fore/aft saddle position, to correct it.

Frame: Measure your inseam from crotch to floor with your bare feet 6 inches apartl; then multiply by 0.65. This equals your road-frame size, measured along the seat tube from the center of the crankset axle to the center of the top tube. As a double check, this should produce 4 to 5 inches of exposed seatpost when your saddle height is correct. (The post's maximum-extension line shouldn't show, of course.) However, remember that a more important dimension is the reach from saddle to handlebar. That's because saddle height is quickly, easily, and inexpensively adjusted, while reach is more difficult to change. Also, many modern road frames use "compact" designs, which feature a sloping top tube, making this formula moot.

Butt: By sliding rearward or forward on the saddle, you can emphasize different muscle groups. This can be useful on a long climb. Moving forward emphasizes the quadriceps muscle, on the fronts of your thighs, while moving back accentuates the opposite side, your hamstrings and glutes.

Feet: Notice your footprints as you walk from a swimming pool. Some of us are pigeon-toed and others are duck-footed. To prevent knee injury, strive for a cleat position that accommodates your natural foot angle. Make cleat adjustments on rides until you feel right, or pay a shop to do it using a fitting device. Better still, use a clipless pedal system that allows your feet to pivot freely ("float"), thus making precise adjustment unnecessary. Position cleats fore/aft so the widest part of each foot is directly above or slightly in front of the pedal axle.

Crankarm length: The trend is toward longer levers. These add power but may inhibit pedaling speed. In general, if your inseam is less than 29 inches, use 165 mm crankarms; if it's from 29 to 32 inches, 170 mm; from 32 to 34 inches, 172.5 mm; and more than 34 inches, 175 mm. Crankarm length is measured from the center of the fixing bolt to the center of the pedal mounting hole. It's usually stamped on the back of the arm.

27 ▶▶▶

MOUNTAIN BIKING POSITION

Frame: Spontaneous (sometimes unwanted) dismounts are a part of riding off-road. Consequently, you need lots of clearance between yourself and the top tube. The ideal mountain bike size is about 4 inches smaller than your road bike size. This isn't as critical if you'll be riding only on pavement or smooth dirt roads, but there's no advantage to having a frame any larger than the smallest size that provides enough saddle height and reach to the handlebar. Smaller frames are lighter, stiffer, and more maneuverable. Because manufacturers specify frame size in different ways, use the stand-over test. When you straddle the bike while wearing your riding shoes, there should be a minimum of 4 inches between your crotch and the top tube.

Saddle height: Seatpost lengths of 350 mm are common, so a lot of post can be out of the frame before the maximum-extension line (etched on the post) shows. For efficient pedaling, your knee should remain slightly bent at the bottom of the pedal stroke (the same as with a road bike). However, you may wish to lower the saddle slightly for rough terrain, enabling yourself to rise so the bike can float beneath you without pounding your crotch. On steep descents, some riders drop the saddle even farther, to keep their weight low and rearward, but others just slide their butts off the back.

Saddle tilt: Most off-road riders prefer a level saddle, but some (including many women) find that a slight nose-down tilt avoids pressure and irritation. Others go slightly nose-up, which helps them sit back and lessens strain on their arms.

Fore/aft saddle position: This variable is not for adjusting your reach to the handlebar—that's why stems come with different extensions. Use the same procedure described for roadies on page 104.

Stem: Mountain bike stems come in a huge variety of extensions (from 60 to 150 mm) and rises (from −5 to +25 degrees). For good control, the stem should place the bar an inch or two below the top of the saddle. This helps put weight on the front wheel so it's easier to steer on climbs and the wheel is less likely to leave the ground. The extension should allow comfortably bent arms and a straight back. A longer and lower reach works for fast cruising, but a higher, closer hand position affords more control on difficult trails. If you're looking for a more upright position, consider a "riser" handlebar, which bends upward as much as 1½ inches.

Handlebar width: An end-to-end measurement of 21 to 24 inches is common. If the bar seems too wide, it can be trimmed with a hacksaw or a pipe cutter. First, though, move your controls and grips inward, and take a ride to make sure you'll like the new width. And remember to leave a bit extra at each end if you use bar ends. In general, the narrower the handlebar, the quicker the steering. Wider bars provide more control at slow speed.

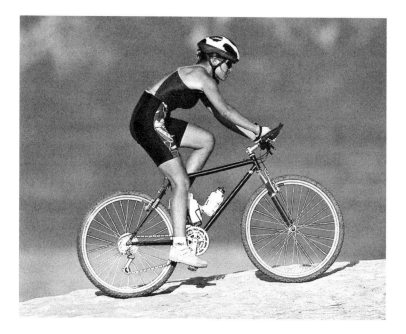

Handlebar sweep: Flat bars can be straight or have up to 11 degrees of rearward bend per side. The choice is strictly one of arm and wrist comfort. Be aware that changing the sweep also changes your reach to the grips and could require a different stem length. Also available are bars with an upward bend or rise. These can allow a lower stem position.

Bar ends: These are great for getting climbing leverage and achieving a longer, lower position on flat fire roads or pavement. Angle them slightly upward. Models that curve inward help protect your hands and are less likely to snag brush on tight singletrack. If you're thinking of installing bar ends, make sure your handlebar can accept them. Some ultralight bars can't.

Crankarm length: Manufacturers usually vary this with frame size. For greater leverage on steep climbs, a mountain bike typically comes with crankarms 5 mm longer than would a road bike for the same size rider.

Arms: Slightly bent arms act as shock absorbers. If you can reach the bar only with straight elbows, get a shorter stem or condition yourself to lean forward more by rotating your hips.

Back: When your top tube/stem length combo is correct, you should have a forward lean of about 45 degrees during normal riding. This is an efficient angle because the strong gluteus muscles of your buttocks don't contribute much to pedaling when you're sitting more upright. Plus, a forward lean shifts some weight to your arms, so your butt doesn't get as sore.

Upper body: Don't hunch your shoulders, and you'll avoid muscle soreness and fatigue. Tilt your head every few minutes to stave off tight neck muscles.

Hands and wrists: Grasp the bar just firmly enough to maintain control. Set the brake levers close to the grips, and angle them so you can extend a finger or two around each and still hold the bar comfortably. Your wrists should be straight when you're standing over the saddle and braking, as on a downhill. Always ride with your thumbs under the bar so your hands can't slip off.

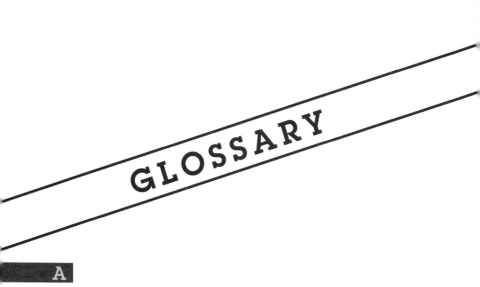

GLOSSARY

A

Aerobic: Exercise at an intensity that allows the body's need for oxygen to be continually met. This intensity can be sustained for long periods.

Anaerobic: Exercise above the intensity at which the body's need for oxygen can be met. This intensity can be sustained only briefly.

Anaerobic threshold (AT): *See* Lactate threshold.

B

Bonk: To run out of energy, usually because the rider has failed to eat or drink enough.

BPM: Abbreviation for "beats per minute" in reference to heart rate.

C

Cadence: The number of times during 1 minute that a pedal stroke is completed. Also called pedal rpm.

Carbohydrate: In the diet, it is broken down to glucose, the body's principal energy source, through digestion and metabolism. Carb can be simple (sugars) or complex (bread, pasta, grains, fruits, vegetables); the latter type contains additional nutrients. One gram of carbohydrate supplies 4 calories.

Century: A ride of 100 miles or 100 kilometers (called a metric century).

Chondromalacia: A softening or wearing away and cracking of the cartilage under the kneecap, resulting in pain and inflammation.

Circuit training: A weight training technique in which you move rapidly from exercise to exercise with no rest.

Criterium: A short-course road race featuring numerous laps with tight turns. It puts a premium on cornering and sprinting ability.

Cross training: Combining sports for mental refreshment and physical conditioning, especially during cycling's off-season.

D

Downshift: to shift to a lower gear—that is, to a larger cog or a smaller chainring.

Draft: The slipstream created by a moving rider. Another rider close behind can keep the same pace using about 30 percent less energy.

E

Ergometer: A stationary device typically found in human-performance labs. It is pedaled like a bicycle and may measure power output in watts. Resistance comes from friction against a large flywheel.

F

Fat: In the diet, it is the most concentrated source of food energy, supplying 9 calories per gram. Stored fat provides about half the energy required for low-intensity exercise.

Fixed gear: A single-speed drivetrain that does not allow coasting. When the bike rolls, the crankset turns. It is used on track bikes and sometimes for early-season road training.

Force: The ability to apply pressure to the pedals.

G

Glutes: The gluteal muscles of the buttocks. They are key to pedaling power.

Glycemic index: The ranking of foods according to their immediate effect on blood glucose levels.

Glycemic load: A measure of the total glycemic response to a food, calculated by multiplying the glycemic index by grams of carbohydrate per serving.

Glycogen: A fuel derived as glucose (sugar) from carbohydrate and stored in the muscles and liver. It's the primary energy source for high-intensity cycling. Reserves are normally depleted after about 2½ hours of riding.

Glycogen window: The period, within an hour after exercise, when depleted muscles are most receptive to restoring their glycogen content. During this time, eating foods or drinking fluids rich in carbohydrate enhances energy stores and recovery.

Granny gear: The lowest gear ratio, combining the small chainring with the largest cassette cog. It's used mainly for very steep climbs.

H

Hamstrings: The muscles on the backs of the thighs, which are not well-developed by cycling.

I

Interval training: A type of workout in which periods of intense effort are alternated with periods of easy effort for recovery.

L

Lactate: *See* Lactic acid.

Lactate threshold (LT): The exertion level at which the body can no longer produce energy aerobically, resulting in the buildup of lactic acid. This is marked by muscle fatigue, pain, and shallow, rapid breathing. The heart rate at which this occurs is termed LTHR. Also called anaerobic threshold (AT).

Lactic acid: A substance formed during anaerobic metabolism when there is incomplete breakdown of glucose. It rapidly produces muscle fatigue and pain. Also called lactate.

M

Max VO₂: The maximum amount of oxygen that can be consumed during all-out exertion. This is a key indicator of a person's potential in cycling and other aerobic sports. It's largely genetically determined but can be improved somewhat by training.

O

Overreaching: A period of hard training that's designed to shock the body into greater fitness.

Overtraining: Long-lasting physical and mental fatigue resulting from the stress of too much work without enough rest.

P

Pedal rpm: *See* Cadence.

Periodization: The process of dividing training into specific phases by weeks or months.

Power: The combination of speed and strength.

Protein: In the diet, it is required for tissue growth and repair. Composed of structural units called amino acids, protein is not a significant energy source unless enough calories and carbohydrate are consumed. One gram of protein equals 4 calories.

Pushing: Pedaling with a relatively slow cadence, using larger gears.

Q

Quadriceps: The muscle group on the fronts of the thighs, which are well-developed by cycling.

R

Repetition: Also called rep. In weight or interval training, each individual exertion. For example, if you press a barbell five times or do a series of five sprints, you are doing five reps.

Resistance trainer: A stationary training device into which the bike is clamped. Pedaling resistance increases with pedaling speed to simulate actual riding. Also known as an indoor, wind, or mag trainer. The last two names are derived from the fan or magnet that creates resistance on the rear wheel.

Rollers: A stationary training device consisting of three or four long cylinders connected by belts. Both bike wheels roll on these cylinders so that balancing is much like actual riding.

S

Set: In weight or interval training, one group of repetitions. For example, if you do eight reps three times, you are doing three sets.

Speed: The ability to accelerate quickly and maintain a very fast cadence for brief periods.

Speedwork: A general term for intervals and other high-velocity training, such as sprints and time trials.

Spinning: Pedaling with a relatively fast cadence using low to moderate gears.

U

Upshift: To shift to a higher gear—that is, to a smaller cog or a larger chainring.

INDEX

Boldface page references indicate photographs. Underscored references indicate boxed text.